PRAISE FOR *BODIE*

"Adrian Shanker and the contributing authors highlight the need for clinicians to up their game when it comes to caring for sexual and gender minority people. *Bodies and Barriers* serves as a guide, with concrete suggestions for developing knowledge, awareness, and skills to provide holistic care for LGBT people from the cradle to the grave. This book is a gem that centers LGBT people's voices, telling providers exactly how they want to be treated. It's time providers listen to and act on these recommendations."

—Jonathan Mathias Lassiter, PhD, coeditor of *Black LGBT Health in the United States: The Intersection of Race, Gender, and Sexual Orientation*

"Now, more than ever, we need *Bodies and Barriers* to shine a spotlight on how and why good health care for LGBTQ people and our families is such a challenge. *Bodies and Barriers* provides a roadmap for all who are ready to fight for health equity—in the doctor's office, in the halls of government, or in the streets."

—Rea Carey, executive director, National LGBTQ Task Force

"These patient and caregiver experiences ring so loudly in today's environment, when we have compelling evidence of a need for widespread practice change, yet the medical establishment remains slow to respond to the calls from those patients and their caregivers, who are asking so boldly—and rightfully—for those changes. *Bodies and Barriers* is a call to action for learners at all levels, in all health fields, to now start creating a future where health equity is the norm and no one is denied the opportunity to thrive."

—Scott Nass, MD, MPA, president of GLMA: Health Professionals Advancing LGBTQ Equality

"***Bodies and Barriers*** **helps LGBT community members understand the way people in the U.S. health services market erect barriers to anyone who is not the source of easy and immediate profit and helps us all confront and break down these barriers. It helps families of LGBT people understand these obstacles and options for getting around them. And it helps health professionals hear the voices of all their patients, so that we learn to listen and how to care for everyone."**

—Michael Fine, MD, former director of the Rhode Island Department of Health and author of *Health Care Revolt: How to Organize, Build a Health Care System, and Resuscitate Democracy—All at the Same Time*

"***Bodies and Barriers*** **is truly a must-read for anyone working in medical care, social services, or public health. This book brings us closer to the goal of patient-centered care, not only for LGBT communities but for everyone."**

—Kristen Emory, PhD, director and advisor at the Undergraduate Program at San Diego State University School of Public Health

"In ***Bodies and Barriers,*** **Adrian Shanker makes the case for culturally responsive care that meets the needs of the LGBT community. Through compelling essays by LGBT health care consumers, this book enables nurses and all health care professionals to understand the challenges of LGBT clients, families, and communities—and is a call to action for everyone involved in patient care to truly listen and learn."**

—Sarah Hexem Hubbard, Esq., executive director of the National Nurse-Led Care Consortium

"***Bodies and Barriers*** **is a must read for mental health clinicians who are providing care to LGBT community members. This book has depth, spirit, and a breadth of information that can transform LGBT health care."**

—Sharon Esther Papo, LCSW, executive director of Diversity Center of Santa Cruz County

Bodies and Barriers

Queer Activists on Health

Edited by Adrian Shanker

Foreword by Rachel L. Levine, MD

Afterword by Kate Kendell

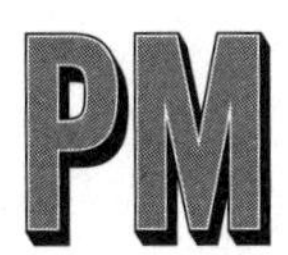

Bodies and Barriers: Queer Activists on Health
Adrian Shanker

This edition published by PM Press

ISBN: 978-1-62963-784-6
Library of Congress Control Number: 2019945894

Section illustrations Jacinta Bunnell
Cover by John Yates / www.stealworks.com
Interior design by briandesign

10 9 8 7 6 5 4 3 2 1

PM Press
PO Box 23912
Oakland, CA 94623
www.pmpress.org
and
The Training Institute at Bradbury-Sullivan LGBT Community Center
522 W. Maple St. *at Bayard Rustin Way*
Allentown, PA 18101
www.bradburysullivancenter.org

Printed in the USA.

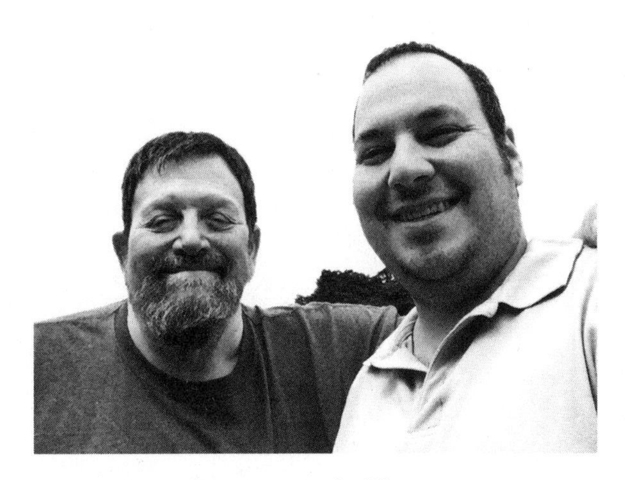

For my cousin Victor,
may his memory be a blessing.
And for queer people everywhere,
whose bodies are prevented from
experiencing health equity
because of all the barriers in the way.
This book is for you.

Contents

Young Adults

Middle-Age Adults

Older Adults

Foreword

Rachel L. Levine, MD

As a physician, I've seen the health consequences of neglecting a patient's needs; as a policy maker, I've seen the cost of creating policies that are uninformed; and as a transgender woman, I've felt the burden of other's ignorance. Too often, LGBT rights are overlooked and set aside as a personal issue for LGBT individuals to tolerate. LGBT rights are irrefutably human rights, and currently there is a significant discrepancy between the treatment of LGBT individuals compared to their heterosexual and cisgender counterparts. The damaging consequences of stripping LGBT individuals of their rights affects far more than just their safety and well-being. LGBT individuals are part of larger communities, families, teams, and social networks. It pains me that these points must be reiterated, however this conversation is clearly pressing and imperative.

As health disparities and social inequities become better understood, the response from health care providers and policy makers must too. LGBT individuals are far more likely to experience poor health outcomes, discrimination, and harassment than the majority population. The 2015 U.S. Transgender Survey indicated that 40 percent of transgender individuals have attempted suicide in their lifetime, nearly nine times the rate of the U.S. population (4.6 percent).[1] Sadly, this is unsurprising. LGBT people face higher rates of violence, including physical attacks, sexual assault, and intimate partner violence. On top of that, LGBT people are less likely to have a support system to confide in.

A quick glimpse of history reveals how these current inequities have manifested. Throughout the years, the criminal justice system has harshly discriminated against the LGBT community. The first documented death penalty for homosexual activity in the United States occurred in 1566, and this continued until the late 1700s.[2] Later, in 1952, the American Psychiatric Association (APA) listed homosexuality as a sociopathic personality disturbance in their diagnostic manual, which only enhanced the stigma surrounding the community and increased discrimination, including in workplaces like the federal government. A year after the APA's classification, President Eisenhower signed an executive order stating that LGBT individuals were a security risk and therefore could not work for the federal government (clearly that didn't last). In 1969, police raided the Stonewall Inn, a bar that was a local hub for the LGBT community in New York City. This raid sparked violent protests that lasted for six days, which ultimately marked a turning point for the LGBT civil rights movement.[3]

The ongoing centuries of persecution and condemnation led to the social movements and pride that exists today. However, we have a long way to go. On June 12, 2016, there was a mass shooting at Pulse Nightclub, a popular gay club in Orlando, that killed forty-nine and injured fifty. This massacre is one of the worst in United States history. The hate that drove this tragic event is not a new phenomenon, but the universal loving response that followed it was. This tragedy revealed the shift in public attitudes toward the LGBT community and reminded us how much more prevalent love is than hate. Since our culture has finally recognized the need to support our LGBT community, it's time that our policies and health care practices do the same.

Comprehensive policies that address discrimination in multiple sectors must be developed to deconstruct centuries of systematic oppression. Currently, there aren't any statewide antidiscrimination protections for LGBT people in twenty-nine states, including Pennsylvania. LGBT individuals can get married on a Friday but could be denied housing on a Saturday, banned from using a public restroom on a Sunday, and fired for their sexual orientation or gender identity on a Monday. To counteract this reality, the Pennsylvania Fairness Act was introduced in the 2015–2016 session and again in the 2017–2018 session. The Act would extend nondiscrimination provisions in state law to protect transgender individuals. However, as I write this, the bill has yet to be brought up for a vote.

Federal protections also seem to be up in the air. Section 1557 of the Patient Protection and Affordable Care Act (ACA) is a nondiscrimination provision that prohibits discrimination based on race, color, origin, sex, age, or ability.[4] This provision is being reconsidered to exclude gender identity protections. In December of 2016, a preliminary injunction was issued to prohibit the Office of Civil Rights (OCR) from enforcing parts of Section 1557 that prevented discrimination based on gender identity.[5]

This policy deficiency is creating wider disparities, and without policy reform, this reality won't change. New policies and practices must be influenced by LGBT individuals to accurately represent their needs. Additionally, health care organizations should adopt policies that require their providers to become more educated in LGBT care.

According to the *2015 U.S. Transgender Survey*, one in three transgender individuals had experienced a negative reaction from a health care provider in the previous year.[6] In Pennsylvania, one in three report their provider is either slightly or not at all competent in LGBT issues, and three in four transgender and gender nonconforming respondents report that they often or always fear a negative reaction by a health care provider.[7] Although I've witnessed society becoming more accepting over the years, lack of awareness and stigma still persists in policy and health care.

I've had the illuminating opportunity to see this reality from both sides. For many years, I practiced adolescent and transgender medicine. I've seen the far-reaching positive outcomes of providing competent care to patients. Some patients I saw for transgender medicine also had mental health conditions like anxiety, depression, post-traumatic stress disorder (PTSD), self-harm, and disordered eating. Having a negative reaction from a health care provider during this time would have been detrimental to their well-being. Additionally, it's vital to the patient's safety that they feel comfortable enough to share information about all medications that they're taking, including hormones, to avoid a negative interaction. I'm aware that treating LGBT patients with multiple conditions can be challenging at times due to parents' influence, social constructs, and lack of experience, but that comes with treating any patient, and it's vital that we provide equitable care to this community.

On the other hand, I can testify to how disheartening it is to seek guidance or care from a provider that is not competent in LGBT care. I've heard many stories of individuals seeking support from a therapist, only to be met with the opposite. Additionally, many patients struggle to find a primary care provider that is competent in LGBT health. This lack of awareness leads to unproductive visits, and ultimately less healthy patients. In this common scenario, it seems like the LGBT community is not valued, and ignorance is acceptable.

The saying is true that we haven't made progress unless we all make progress. Within the LGBT community, some individuals are more likely to experience specific disparities based on their sexual orientation or gender identity. For example, 46 percent of bisexual women have been victims of rape, compared to 13 percent of lesbians.[8] Additionally, Black/African American transgender individuals are more likely to have HIV diagnoses than their White or Hispanic/Latino counterparts.[9] It's vital that providers become educated on these specific disparities, so that they we can leverage this information to address the unique concerns of these groups.

The multidimensional degree of systematic inequalities calls for significant action among health care providers and policy makers. It's unacceptable for providers and policy makers to continue to turn a shoulder to this issue.

As you read through the following texts, I challenge you to let these stories resonate with you and to let them influence your perception. Consider where you play into the solution and how you can use any ounce of privilege that you have to advocate for LGBT health. LGBT individuals deserve to live happy and healthy lives, and that liberty begins with us listening.

Rachel L. Levine, MD, is the secretary of health for the Commonwealth of Pennsylvania and professor of pediatrics and psychiatry at the Pennsylvania State College of Medicine. She is a fellow of the American Academy of Pediatrics, the Society for Adolescent Health and Medicine, and the Academy for Eating Disorders. She is a member of the World Professional Association for Transgender Health. She is also a board member and executive committee member of the Association of State and Territorial Health Officials. Dr. Levine joined Governor Tom Wolf's administration in January 2015 as the physician general of the Commonwealth of Pennsylvania and served from 2015 to 2017. Upon her appointment, she became the first transgender person to hold a cabinet position in Pennsylvania. In 2017, she was named the acting secretary of health, and in 2018 she was confirmed by the Pennsylvania Senate as the secretary of health. She leads the LGBTQ Policy Workgroup and advocates for LGBTQ rights for the Wolf administration. Dr. Levine is also an accomplished regional and international speaker and author on the opioid crisis, medical marijuana, adolescent medicine, eating disorders, and LGBT medicine. Dr. Levine graduated from Harvard College and the Tulane University School of Medicine. She completed her training in pediatrics and adolescent medicine at the Mount Sinai Medical Center in New York City.

Notes

1. S.E. James, J.L. Herman, S. Rankin, M. Keisling, L. Mottet, and M. Anafi, *2015 U.S. Transgender Survey* (Washington, DC: National Center for Transgender Equality, 2016), accessed May 31, 2019, https://transequality.org/sites/default/files/docs/usts/USTS-Full-Report-Dec17.pdf.
2. Bonnie J. Morris, "History of Lesbian, Gay, Bisexual and Transgender Social Movements," American Psychological Association, accessed May 31, 2019, https://www.apa.org/pi/lgbt/resources/history.aspx; GSAFE, "A Timeline of Lesbian, Gay, Bisexual, and Transgender History in the United States," accessed May 31, 2019, https://www.gsafewi.org/wp-content/uploads/US-LGBT-Timeline-UPDATED.pdf.
3. Morris, "History of Lesbian, Gay, Bisexual and Transgender Social Movements."
4. United States Department of Health and Human Services, "Section 1557 of the Patient Protection and Affordable Care Act," HSS.gov Civil Rights, 2018, accessed May 31, 2019, https://www.hhs.gov/civil-rights/for-individuals/section-1557/index.html.
5. Katie Keith, "More Courts Rule on Section 1557 as HHS Reconsiders Regulation," *Health Affairs*, October 2, 2018, accessed May 31, 2019, www.healthaffairs.org/do/10.1377/hblog20181002.142178/full/.
6. James et al., *2015 U.S. Transgender Survey*.
7. Pennsylvania Department of Health, Division of Tobacco Prevention and Control, *Pennsylvania 2018 LGBT Health Needs Assessment—Summary Report*, August 2018, accessed May 31, 2019, www.livehealthypa.com/docs/default-source/toolkits/lgbt/2018-pa-lgbt-needs-assessment.pdf?sfvrsn=0.
8. "Sexual Assault and the LGBTQ Community," Human Rights Campaign, accessed May 31, 2019, https://www.hrc.org/resources/sexual-assault-and-the-lgbt-community.
9. "HIV among Transgender People," Centers for Disease Control and Prevention, updated April 16, 2019, accessed May 31, 2019, https://www.cdc.gov/hiv/group/gender/transgender/index.html.

Introduction

Adrian Shanker

I am a full-time queer activist leading an LGBT community-based nonprofit organization with a focus on LGBT health equity, and it happened to me too.

By "it," I mean a negative experience with a health care professional because of my queer identity.

I made an appointment with a dermatologist for a baseline screening for skin cancer. But at every turn the doctor's well-intentioned team made me question if I should be there at all. The intake forms were unnecessarily restrictive, biased news programming was on full-display in the waiting room, magazines in the waiting room did not cater to patients like me, and comments from the clinic staff displayed brazen cultural incompetence. I didn't go back for the doctor-recommended follow-up.

I'm privileged with health insurance, access to private transportation, and the ability to take time away from my job to drive a distance for a medical appointment, so I was able to find a new LGBT-inclusive dermatologist an hour away. For many other LGBT consumers of health care, the geographic barrier to accessing culturally appropriate LGBT-inclusive care from a specialist might be too great a barrier to overcome.

When I was a graduate student at George Washington University in their LGBT Health Policy & Practice program, I was struck by the lack of literature written by health care consumers and activists to inform health care professionals, students in health professions, and policy makers about the unique health needs faced by the LGBT patient population.

There's a great deal of literature about LGBT health (to be sure, there are still many gaps) but most of it is written *by* researchers or health care professionals *about* LGBT patients. While this literature still adds valuable information, sometimes leading to important behavioral, clinical, or policy changes, LGBT people deserve to write our own narratives. *Our* stories about *our* bodies and the barriers to care *we* experience deserve to directly impact the landscape of care in every community. That's what this book is about.

Throughout our lives, LGBT people experience unique structural barriers to care that lead to higher behavioral risk factors for numerous sexually transmitted and chronic diseases. When compounded with past negative experiences in health care settings, including outright discrimination, the LGBT community experiences worse health outcomes than the majority population.

This isn't our fault. HIV activist Sean Strub (featured in chapter 18) says, "stigma is about other people making a moral judgment about your worth."[1] LGBT people have culturally experienced decades of stigma. In *The History of Sexuality*, vol. 1, Michel Foucault discusses the medical categorization of homosexuality, citing Carl Westphal's 1870 article, "Archiv für Neurologie." Foucault wrote, "it was transposed from the practice of sodomy onto a kind of interior androgyny, a hermaphrodism of the soul. The sodomite had been a temporary aberration; the homosexual was now a species." The medical establishment was looking for a medical "cure" to what was an illegal practice in much of Europe in the 1800s. Foucault continued, "since sexuality was a medical and medicalizable object, one had to try to detect it—as a lesion, a dysfunction, or a symptom—in the depths of the organism or on the surface of the skin, or among all the signs of behavior."[2] Throughout the following decades, the medical establishment came up with many "solutions," some of which included chemical castration, frontal lobotomies, and electroshock therapy, all of which would be considered extreme versions of today's so-called "conversion therapy." Decades of discrimination followed.

In 1976, three years after the American Psychiatric Association removed the diagnosis of "homosexuality" from its *Diagnostic and Statistical Manual* (DSM), Dr. Henry Kazal published an article in the *Annals of Clinical and Laboratory Science* naming a series of unrelated viruses and infections "gay bowel syndrome." This represented the first time an identity group was named as a "syndrome." Kazal wrote "the male homosexual patients seen in a proctologic practice in New York

City presented with a pattern of multiple proctologic diseases which the authors have called the gay bowel syndrome. In the absence of a history of homosexuality, the physician may be alerted to the gay bowel syndrome by anal condyloma . . . [the occurrence of venereal diseases] is attributed to the common promiscuity of gay males and the many opportunities for fecal-oral contact. The cases were scattered with no suggestion of epidemic spread. These patients could be a public health hazard if employed as food handlers."[3] Among the problems with Kazal's research was that there is nothing biological among gay males leading to increased risk for any of the viruses or infections he categorized within "gay bowel syndrome." The risk factors are based on behaviors not exclusive to gay men but exacerbated due to social and cultural experiences with discrimination, harassment, bullying, family rejection, and violence, compounded by a lack of culturally appropriate, comprehensive sex education.

In response to Kazal, Michael Scarce published a 2002 article in the *International Journal of Epidemiology*, facetiously coining "heterocopulative syndrome." He wrote, "The hazards of heterosexual behaviour have been well documented. They include, but are not limited to, unplanned pregnancies, penile and cervical cancer, vaginitis, a host of sexually transmitted diseases (some of them incurable or deadly), a disproportionate propensity to engage in child molestation, global overpopulation, socially oppressive gender roles, and more. A recurring pattern of these health disorders resulting from the union of the penis and vagina has been named heterocopulative syndrome. These people could pose a serious public health threat if such practices continue unchecked and may be especially dangerous if employed as food handlers."[4]

A fourteen-year-old youth program participant at Whitman-Walker Health Clinic in Washington, DC, shared that "wellness is about surviving in a world that was not created for you." That's what the LGBT patient population has been bravely doing for decades. Surviving conversion therapy. Surviving family rejection. Surviving discrimination. And, to be sure, not everyone survived, not by a long shot. No book on LGBT health is complete without an acknowledgement of the pain—the loss of a generation to AIDS, the loss of forty-nine queer lives at Pulse Nightclub, the loss of so many queer bodies to homicide, suicide, substance overdose, and hate crimes. And with the acknowledgment of pain, we must also acknowledge that survival is a privilege. That the chances of surviving are higher for white, higher income, cisgender men.

Those who survive our unfair landscape persevere through barriers at every step of the way—barriers created by the government, by the medical establishment, by the pharmaceutical industry, and by insurance companies. We live with increased tobacco, alcohol, and other drug usage. We live with increased risk for obesity and diabetes. We live with increased risk for chronic diseases, including HIV and cancer. We live with increased discrimination, violence, harassment, and bullying. We live with family rejection and minority stress. And we are demanding that our health care systems respond to our lived experiences with culturally appropriate care at all stages of our lives.

This book is arranged to follow the lifespan—youth, young adults, middle-age adults, and older adults. Every health care professional can benefit from this book. From those who work in labor and delivery to those who provide hospice care. From primary care clinicians to specialists in every health field. From surgeons and family doctors to nurses, counselors, social workers, and pharmacists. Every person providing care for humans is providing care for LGBT humans.

Likewise, every health policy maker can benefit from this book. From legislative and executive branch public officials to insurance regulators and health network administrators, the policies made by public and private institutions directly impact health outcomes for the LGBT patient population. Every person involved in health policy making is making policy that affects LGBT people.

Finally, every activist for the LGBT community can benefit from this book. From emerging activists to nonprofit leaders, from pride organizers to those engaged in direct action, the activism that supports the LGBT community improves our health. This book will demonstrate that what is defined as health is broad, and that our health in inseparable from all other aspects of our lives. When activists for the LGBT community incorporate health care frameworks into our work, we can broaden our coalitions and increase support for legal and social change.

Essays included in this book represent diverse identities within the LGBT community, and no author can claim to represent the entire LGBT community. When you've heard from one of us, you've heard from exactly one of us. LGBT health challenges differ for urban and rural communities. They differ between countries, states, provinces, and territories. They differ across our diverse identities, abilities, and generations within the LGBT community. They differ based on family support and many other factors. What is clear throughout the diverse LGBT community is that we, as a historically underrepresented and marginalized population, experience severe and pervasive health disparities, and we experience them throughout our bodies and throughout our lives.

My hope is that this text will provide increased understanding of some of the unique challenges LGBT people experience and will lead to an increased prioritization for behavioral, clinical, and policy changes to eliminate LGBT health disparities and improve LGBT health outcomes. As you read the essays in this book, consider how you can improve LGBT health outcomes through behavioral, clinical, or policy lenses.

LGBT people lack health equity, defined by the United States Department of Health and Human Services as "the attainment of the highest levels of health for all people."[5] Our queer bodies deserve health equity. Together, let us tear down the barriers to care so we can achieve it.

Notes

1 Sean Strub, "HIV Community Empowerment," B Stigma Free (blog), accessed May 31, 2019, http://bstigmafree.org/blog/hiv-community-empowerment/.

2 Michel Foucault, *The History of Sexuality, vol. 1: An Introduction* (New York: Vintage Books, 1990). 43–44.

3 Henry L. Kazal, Norman Sohn, Jose I. Carrasco, James G. Robilotti, Jr., and William E. Delaney, "The Gay Bowel Syndrome: Clinico-Pathologic Correlation in 260 Cases," *Annals of Clinical and Laboratory Science* 6, no. 2 (March–April 1976): 184–92, accessed May 31, 1019, www.annclinlabsci.org/content/6/2/184.full.pdf.

4 Michael Scarce, "Heterocopulative Syndrome: Clinico-Pathologic Correlation in 260 Cases," *International Journal of Epidemiology* 31, no. 2 (April 2002): 498–99, accessed May 31, 2019, https://academic.oup.com/ije/article/31/2/498/2951449.

5 United States Department of Health and Human Services, Office of Disease Prevention and Health Promotion, "Lesbian, Gay, Bisexual, and Transgender Health," Healthy People 2020, accessed May 31, 2019, https://www.healthypeople.gov/2020/topics-objectives/topic/lesbian-gay-bisexual-and-transgender-health.

A Note on Terminology

The LGBT community is not one but many communities. Through our diversity of generations, geographies, gender identities, sexual orientations, races, and abilities, language is not constant. For the purpose of consistency, this book uses the acronym "LGBT." We do so with recognition that there are a multiplicity of additional letters representing identities sometimes further marginalized within the LGBT community.

We also use the word "queer" when appropriate in the text. Some authors in this text and some readers may find this word objectionable. If an author objected to the word "queer," it is not used in their chapter. The word "queer" is used positively to affirm social, political, and sexual difference and a desire to live outside of societal expectations of normativity. It has historically also been used as a dehumanizing epithet. For readers who are new to seeing the word "queer" used in a positive space, understand that for those of us who claim "queer" as our identity, we do so with pride and intention but also be aware that it is unwise to assume that all LGBT people will want to be referred to as "queer." Health care professionals should mirror the language their patients use to describe their own identities.

A Note on Section Header Illustrations

Hand-drawn section headers in this book are the work of queer, feminist coloring book artist Jacinta Bunnell (*Girls Are Not Chicks; Girls Will Be Boys Will Be Girls Will Be. . .*). These pages offer coloring breaks for our readers. Go ahead, break the rules, color outside the lines!

Acknowledgments

An edited text is only as good as the content included in it, so a heartfelt thank you to each of the contributing authors—all of whom inspire me to keep fighting every day for queer health. And with special gratitude to Rachel L. Levine, MD, and Kate Kendell—who have both accomplished so much progress for the LGBT community—for their respective foreword and afterword.

Thank you to the entire team at PM Press, especially Steven Stothard and Michael Ryan, John Yates of Stealworks for designing the book cover, and Jacinta Bunnell for so beautifully illustrating the section headers throughout the book. A special thank you to Liz Bradbury, Carolyn Burns, Anthony Crisci, Laura Fassbender, Patrick Fligge, Vipul Shukla, Bennett Urian, and my grandfather Ronald Levant for their support and advice throughout the process of creating this book.

Bodies and Barriers was edited during a sabbatical made possible by the board of directors of Bradbury-Sullivan LGBT Community Center, with support from the Lehigh Valley Community Foundation. Many thanks to my longtime friend Kim Nguyen, my gracious sabbatical host, and Adrian Khactu, who, along with Kim, made me feel at home in a faraway place.

And to the incredible team at Bradbury-Sullivan LGBT Community Center—who *show up* for queer health equity day in and day out—*I am proud to work alongside you to promote high-quality health for our community.*

YOUTH

Human Rights and Health for LGBT Youth

Ryan Thoreson

Introduction

Health interventions for LGBT youth are typically framed in medical not legal terms. But a human rights perspective offers a powerful tool to address health disparities and improve outcomes for LGBT youth. A human right is a right that all people, regardless of their background or citizenship, possess simply because they are human. When something is recognized as a human right, states are obligated to respect, protect, and promote that right. Health is related to human rights in two distinctive ways. First, the right to health is itself a human right, enshrined in a wide range of human rights treaties and affirmed by countries around the globe. The Universal Declaration of Human Rights, adopted by the United States and other states at the United Nations after the horrors of World War II, recognizes the right to a standard of living adequate for health and well-being. This right is affirmed in treaties like the International Covenant on Economic, Social and Cultural Rights, the Convention on the Rights of the Child, and the Convention on the Elimination of All Forms of Discrimination Against Women. And, second, the promotion and protection of human rights can improve health by discouraging violence and discrimination, minimizing stressors, and empowering people to voice their needs and seek out resources.

A rights respecting approach is important to improving health outcomes for LGBT youth. By canvassing some of the health disparities that LGBT youth experience, we are able to discuss human rights violations that can contribute to those disparities and explore some of the reasons that promoting human rights can help improve health outcomes. Respecting the rights of LGBT youth is not only a legal obligation or a way to convey affirmation and support. It is also a crucial strategy to improve LGBT youth's health and well-being, with positive effects that can last throughout their lives.

Health Disparities among LGBT Youth

Researchers have identified a range of physical and mental health issues that LGBT youth are more likely to experience than their heterosexual, cisgender peers. These health disparities are avoidable—they are created and exacerbated by conditions that put LGBT youth at risk and make it more difficult for them to obtain care.

The physical health disparities that LGBT youth encounter may not be as pronounced as those that LGBT adults might face later in their lives, but they can still be evident from an early age. In 2017, the U.S. government collected nationally representative data on health and well-being from students in grades nine to twelve, including questions about sexual identity. In that study, 21.9 percent of LGB students reported that they had been physically forced to have sexual intercourse against their will in the year before the survey—nearly four times the rate of heterosexual students. Similarly, 22.2 percent of LGB students had experienced sexual violence—defined as being forced to do sexual acts they did not want to do—at almost three times the rate of heterosexual students. In dating and relationships too LGB youth reported significantly higher rates of sexual dating violence and physical dating violence.[1] Data collection is more limited for transgender youth, but federal data released in 2019 indicate that 23.8 percent had been forced to have sexual intercourse and 26.4 percent had experienced physical dating violence in the year prior to the survey and had faced higher rates of violence than cisgender youth.[2] From a sexual health perspective, LGBT youth are at heightened risk of HIV and sexually transmitted infections compared to their peers. In 2016, young gay and bisexual men made up 81 percent of new HIV diagnoses among youth in the United States, with particularly high infection rates among young Black, Latino, and/or bisexual men.[3] Data suggest transgender youth are less likely to have been tested for HIV than their cisgender peers.[4]

Evidence suggests that LGB youth are also less likely to be physically active than their heterosexual counterparts. In federal data from 2017, LGB students consistently reported lower rates of physical activity, participation in team sports, and attendance in physical education classes and were more likely to play video or computer games or watch television more than three hours a day.[5] LGB youth were also slightly more likely to be obese or overweight—and more likely to perceive themselves as overweight and be trying to lose weight—than heterosexual youth.[6]

Moreover, LGBT youth are more likely than their heterosexual, cisgender peers to engage in behaviors that jeopardize health. LGBT youth consistently demonstrate higher rates of alcohol, tobacco, and other drug use, and research shows these disparities persist into adulthood.[7] In data collected in 2017, students questioning their sexual orientations were even more likely than LGB students to have used cocaine, inhalants, heroin, methamphetamines, hallucinogenic drugs, and injection drugs, though both groups used these drugs—as well as synthetic marijuana, ecstasy, and prescription painkillers—at higher rates than heterosexual students.[8] In federal data on substance abuse, transgender youth were more likely than cisgender youth to have used every substance listed except marijuana.[9]

Yet disparities are particularly pronounced in the field of mental health. While many LGBT youth do not struggle with mental health issues, research has powerfully shown that LGB youth as a population are at an elevated risk of depression, anxiety, and suicidality.[10] In keeping with these factors, researchers have noted that a "higher risk for suicide ideation attempts among LGB groups seems to start at least as early as high school."[11] While data has been more limited for transgender youth, existing research suggests they also experience disproportionately high rates of depression, eating disorders, self-harm, and suicidal ideation and behavior.[12]

Disparities in physical and mental health are neither inevitable nor intractable. In many cases, laws, policies, and practices that restrict human rights have demonstrably negative effects on LGBT youth health. A rights respecting approach to LGBT issues in youth can help to advance a range of human rights—including the right to the highest attainable standard of physical and mental health.

Human Rights Violations Faced by LGBT Youth

The persistence of health disparities has led researchers to examine why, holding other demographic and environmental factors equal, LGBT youth tend to be at higher risk of worsened health outcomes. One key finding in recent years is that human rights violations, as well as more subtle and persistent forms of marginalization, can play a powerful role in generating or exacerbating the health risks that youth face.

Among the most common issues that LGBT youth experience are bullying and harassment, which too often go unchecked by staff. In interviews I conducted in 2015, Alexander S., a sixteen-year-old transgender boy in Texas, described how he had been verbally and physically bullied since elementary school for his gender expression and began suffering from depression and suicidal thoughts from a young age. When he turned to teachers and the school and they failed to intervene, he kept the persistent harassment to himself.[13]

Unfortunately, Alexander's story is one of many. According to federal data collected in 2017, one-third of gay, lesbian, and bisexual students had been bullied on school property in the year before the survey, compared to 17.1 percent of heterosexual students.[14] According to GLSEN's National School Climate Survey in 2017, verbal harassment is also common, with 70.1 percent of LGBT students experiencing harassment based on their sexual orientation and 59.1 percent experiencing harassment based on their gender identity.[15] Verbal harassment is not only at the hands of peers; 56.6 percent of students had heard homophobic remarks and 71.0 percent had heard transphobic remarks from teachers or staff.[16] According to federal data collected in 2017, LGB students experienced cyberbullying at more than double the rate of heterosexual students who reported similar experiences.[17] In qualitative interviews, LGBT students have reported being targeted for cyberbullying because of their gender or sexuality, being catfished with fake dating profiles, or being intentionally misgendered online as a form of humiliation.[18] Despite these alarming statistics, only twenty states and the District of Columbia have laws prohibiting bullying on the basis of sexual orientation and gender identity.[19]

The health of transgender youth is also directly compromised by discriminatory policies that do not recognize their gender identity. Susanna K., the mother of a transgender boy in Utah, told me that her son began suffering from bladder infections in junior high, and that she eventually discovered that it was because he did not feel safe in male or female bathrooms at school. When she enrolled him at a charter school that respected his gender identity, the bladder infections stopped. When transgender students are required to use bathrooms and other facilities according to their sex assigned at birth, they are highly vulnerable to harassment and assault. Many transgender students thus avoid using these facilities at all. Students have described how they limit fluid intake or wait until the school day ends to relieve themselves, which can lead to dehydration, bladder infections, urinary tract infections, and other health complications.[20] When transgender students generally are not allowed to participate in sports and other extracurriculars consistent with their gender identity—a rule adopted by nine US states—they frequently forego participation in athletics, depriving them of the physical, mental, and social benefits that other youth enjoy.[21]

One of the ways that LGBT youth have traditionally found support is through the formation of gay-straight alliances or other LGBT student groups. For many LGBT youth, participation in an LGBT student group is essential to reducing feelings of social isolation and accessing information. Schools that have attempted to deny registration to these groups or that have created unfair burdens, such as requiring parental notification for students to participate, have been stopped by federal courts, which have found that these groups must be treated on the same terms as all other extracurricular student organizations. Nonetheless, research suggests that schools across the country still interfere with the formation or operation of LGBT student groups, by dragging out their registration, imposing requirements on those groups that they do not impose on other student organizations, monitoring their meetings, or prohibiting them from discussing certain topics. Such restrictions not only violate LGBT students' freedom of expression, assembly, and association but prevent LGBT students from forming communities that alleviate isolation, bolster self-esteem, and affirm their identities.

The use of conversion therapy, whether on the basis of sexual orientation or gender identity, has also been recognized as a human rights violation—in some instances, a form of torture. Practices of conversion therapy can threaten physical health, for example, when practitioners use aversive therapy to physically punish any sign of interest in same-sex activity. These practices can also threaten mental health. According to the American Psychological Association, conversion therapy can produce negative effects like "anger, anxiety, confusion, depression, grief, guilt, hopelessness, deteriorated relationships with family, loss of social support, loss of faith, poor self-image, social isolation, intimacy difficulties, intrusive imagery, suicidal ideation, self-hatred, and sexual dysfunction."[22] Refusing to recognize trans youth can also exacerbate gender dysphoria and related forms of psychological distress. When trans youth who want to physically transition are denied access to transition-related care, they may seek out alternatives, including black market hormones, silicone, and unsupervised modifications to their bodies with potentially serious and lasting repercussions for their health.

Rejection can impair health in slightly more attenuated ways as well. In large part because of family rejection, LGBT youth are at a significantly higher risk of homelessness than their heterosexual, cisgender peers. In 2012, the Williams Institute estimated that LGBT youth made up about 40 percent of homeless youth in the United States—a disproportionately high figure relative to the percentage of LGBT youth in the population overall.[23] Failing to protect LGBT youth from homelessness not only deprives them of the right to adequate housing but puts them at heightened risk of other human rights violations, including violations of their physical and mental health.

Silence around LGBT issues can also exacerbate health disparities. While many youth in the United States lack access to comprehensive sexuality education, that absence is especially acute for LGBT youth. It is extremely rare for LGBT youth to receive information about safer sex that pertains to their needs. In six states, laws specifically prohibit discussions of same-sex activity in sexuality education classes—a policy that often has a chilling effect across the school curriculum.[24] Such policies, like filtering out age-appropriate LGBT content on school computers or banning LGBT books from school libraries, unduly restrict LGBT youth's right to access information as well as their right to health.

Other forms of discrimination jeopardize LGBT well-being as well. In some instances, LGBT youth are unable to bring their partners to school dances or are punished for displays of affection that teachers ignore with their heterosexual, cisgender peers. In some cases, transgender youth have been required to adhere to a gender-based dress code for yearbook photos or graduation and have been forced to wear clothing that is in opposition to their gender identity. Discrimination is overtly codified for many transgender youth, who are unable to use their names and pronouns, wear clothing conforming with their gender identity, access school facilities, or otherwise be themselves in school environments. Without support, these suggestions that LGBT youth are invalid or unwelcome can adversely affect their mental health and sense of belonging in schools.

Even for youth who are not directly subjected to physical or psychological violence, more ambient forms of alienation and stigmatization can shape health outcomes. One way that marginalization can adversely affect LGBT youth is through the cumulative effects of minority stress. Psychologists have developed the concept of minority stress "to distinguish the excess stress to which individuals from stigmatized social categories are exposed as a result of their social, often a minority, position."[25] A 2011 report from the Institute of Medicine similarly underscored that "the disparities in both mental and physical health that are seen between LGBT and heterosexual and non-gender-variant youth are influenced largely by their experiences of stigma and discrimination during the development of their sexual orientation and gender identity and throughout the life course."[26] Such stress can be acutely felt by LGBT youth, who are often in the early stages of exploring their sexual orientation or gender identity, grapple with stigma, lack support from family, friends, or community, have few LGBT role models, or find it difficult to create or access supportive spaces where they can meet and interact with other LGBT people.

As these examples show, much of the distress that LGBT youth experience is preventable. And in addition to stopping bad practices, supporters of LGBT youth can—and should—take concrete steps to respect their rights and affirm their identities.

Resilience and Support

While most research on LGBT youth has focused on health disparities and violations that exacerbate them, recent work has also explored how rights respecting initiatives can mitigate disparities between LGBT youth and their heterosexual, cisgender peers to improve health outcomes. As this research shows, LGBT youth are not inherently doomed to experience poor health; affirming interventions can make a measurable difference in their health and well-being. To advance a more rights respecting paradigm, it is worth describing some of the ways that advocates and providers might support LGBT youth in their work.

For any adults who might work with LGBT youth, research suggests that affirmation can have a positive effect on health outcomes. A supportive environment has been linked to better physical and mental health among LGBT youth, including lower levels of depression, hopelessness, substance use, and suicidality.[27] Affirming transgender youth in the process of social transition has also been associated with better mental health outcomes.[28] In one study that examined the use of chosen names at home, at school, at work, and with friends, for example, researchers found that transgender youth who could use their chosen names in a wider range of contexts were less likely to report depressive symptoms and suicidal ideation or behavior.[29]

Schools can also improve outcomes in a variety of ways. In addition to passing nondiscrimination and anti-bullying protections, schools can ensure that staff are trained to intervene in bullying and harassment, promulgate curricula that speak to LGBT experiences, incorporate LGBT content into libraries and information resources, make students aware of safe spaces where they can discuss stressors, and cultivate and support LGBT student groups. Schools should be aware that students may have difficulty creating or sustaining LGBT student groups, particularly in smaller schools or rural areas. Every effort should be made to support them in doing so, including partnerships with other schools in the area to create a critical mass of students for regular meetings and events.

Finally, lawmakers also have a role to play. Research suggests that expressly prohibiting discrimination based on sexual orientation and gender identity may improve health outcomes. Laws that explicitly prohibit bullying on the basis of sexual orientation, for example, have been associated with lower rates of bullying, fewer stressors, and fewer suicide attempts.[30] Unfortunately, many lawmakers have continued to push policies that do the opposite and consistently target transgender youth for discriminatory treatment. Abandoning efforts to restrict the rights of LGBT youth in favor of a rights respecting approach is an important first step in eradicating the more persistent health disparities that LGBT youth face.

Conclusion

LGBT youth face unique health challenges, many of which have lasting consequences throughout their lives. A rights respecting approach is essential to any effective response to these issues. Protecting the rights of LGBT youth not only shields them from immediate physical and mental harm but takes them out of situations where they are especially vulnerable and equips them with the knowledge, confidence, and resources to protect their health and seek out resources when they are needed.

Ryan Thoreson is the Cover-Lowenstein Fellow in International Human Rights at Yale Law School and a researcher in the LGBT Rights Program at Human Rights Watch. He holds a JD from Yale Law School, a D.Phil. in Anthropology from Oxford University, where he was a Rhodes Scholar, and an AB in Government and Studies of Women, Gender, and Sexuality from Harvard University. He is the author of *Transnational LGBT Activism: Working for Sexual Rights Worldwide.*

Notes

1 Centers for Disease Control and Prevention, "Youth Risk Behavior Surveillance—United States, 2017," *Morbidity and Mortality Weekly Report Surveillance Summaries* 67, no. 8 (2018): 1–114, accessed June 7, 2019, https://www.cdc.gov/mmwr/volumes/67/ss/ss6708a1.htm.
2 Michelle M. Johns, Richard Lowry, Jack Andrzejewski, Lisa C. Barrios; Zewditu Demissie, Timothy McManus, Catherine N. Rasberry, Leah Robin, and J. Michael Underwood (Centers for Disease Control and Prevention), "Transgender Identity and Experiences of Violence Victimization, Substance Use, Suicide Risk, and Sexual Risk Behaviors Among High School Students—19 States and Large Urban School Districts, 2017," *Morbidity and Mortality Weekly Report*, January 25, 2019, 2019, 67–71, accessed June 1, https://www.cdc.gov/mmwr/volumes/68/wr/mm6803a3.htm.
3 "HIV and Youth," Centers for Disease Control and Prevention, updated April 2019, accessed June 1, 2019, https://www.cdc.gov/hiv/pdf/group/age/youth/cdc-hiv-youth.pdf.
4 Johns et al., "Transgender Identity and Experiences of Violence Victimization."
5 Centers for Disease Control and Prevention, "Youth Risk Behavior Surveillance."
6 Ibid.
7 Ibid.; see also Ethan Mereish, "Addressing Research Gaps in Sexual and Gender Minority Adolescents' Substance Use and Misuse," *Journal of Adolescent Health* 62, no. 6 (June 2018): 645–46, accessed June 1, 2019, https://www.jahonline.org/article/S1054-139X(18)30122-8/fulltext.
8 Centers for Disease Control and Prevention, "Youth Risk Behavior Surveillance."
9 Johns et al., "Transgender Identity and Experiences of Violence Victimization."
10 "'Like Walking Through a Hailstorm': Discrimination against LGBT Youth in US Schools," Human Rights Watch, December 7, 2016, accessed June 1, 2019, https://www.hrw.org/report/2016/12/07/walking-through-hailstorm/discrimination-against-lgbt-youth-us-schools.
11 Ilan H. Meyer, "Prejudice, Social Stress, and Mental Health in Lesbian, Gay, and Bisexual Populations: Conceptual Issues and Research Evidence," *Psychological Bulletin* 129, no. 5 (2003): 674–97, accessed June 1, 2019, https://www.ncbi.nlm.nih.gov/pmc/articles/PMC2072932/.
12 Maureen D. Connolly, Marcus J. Zervos, Charles J. Barone II, Christine C. Johnson, and Christine L.M. Joseph, "The Mental Health of Transgender Youth: Advances in Understanding," *Journal of Adolescent Health* 59, no. 5 (November 2016): 489–95, accessed June 1, 2019, https://www.ncbi.nlm.nih.gov/pubmed/27544457;

Amaya Perez-Brumer, Jack K. Day, Stephen T. Russell, and Mark L. Hatzenbuehler, "Prevalence and Correlates of Suicidal Ideation among Transgender Youth in California: Findings from a Representative, Population-Based Sample of High School Students," *Journal of the American Academy of Child and Adolescent Psychiatry* 56, no. 9 (September 2017): 739–46, accessed June 1, 2019, https://www.ncbi.nlm.nih.gov/pubmed/28838578.

13 "Like Walking Through a Hailstorm."

14 Centers for Disease Control and Prevention, "Youth Risk Behavior Surveillance."

15 Joseph G. Kosciw, Emily A. Greytak, Adrian D. Zongrone, Caitlin M. Clark, and Nhan L. Truong, *The 2017 National School Climate Survey: The Experiences of Lesbian, Gay, Bisexual, Transgender, and Queer Youth in Our Nation's Schools* (New York: GLSEN, 2018).

16 Perez-Brumer et al., "Prevalence and Correlates of Suicidal Ideation among Transgender Youth in California."

17 Centers for Disease Control and Prevention, "Youth Risk Behavior Surveillance."

18 "Like Walking Through a Hailstorm."

19 "Safe Schools Laws: Anti-Bullying," Movement Advancement Project, 2019, accessed June 1, 2019, http://www.lgbtmap.org/equality-maps/safe_school_laws.

20 "Shut Out: Restrictions on Bathroom and Locker Room Access for Transgender Youth in US Schools," Human Rights Watch, September 14, 2016, accessed June 1, 2019, https://www.hrw.org/report/2016/09/14/shut-out/restrictions-bathroom-and-locker-room-access-transgender-youth-us-schools.

21 "Special Addition," TransAthlete, 2019, accessed June 1, 2019, https://www.transathlete.com/k-12.

22 Judith M. Glassgold, Lee Beckstead, Jack Drescher, Beverly Greene, Robin Lin Miller, Roger L. Worthington, and Clinton W. Anderson, *Report of the American Psychological Association Task Force on Appropriate Therapeutic Responses to Sexual Orientation* (Washington, DC: American Psychological Association, 2009).

23 Laura Durso and Gary Gates, *Serving Our Youth: Findings from a National Survey of Service Providers Working with Lesbian, Gay, Bisexual and Transgender Youth Who Are Homeless or at Risk of Becoming Homeless* (Los Angeles: Williams Institute, 2012).

24 "Like Walking Through a Hailstorm."

25 Meyer, "Prejudice, Social Stress, and Mental Health in Lesbian, Gay, and Bisexual Populations."

26 Institute of Medicine, *The Health of Lesbian, Gay, Bisexual, and Transgender People* (Washington, DC: National Academies Press, 2011).

27 Elizabeth A. McConnell, Michelle Birkett, and Brian Mustanski. "Families Matter: Social Support and Mental Health Trajectories Among Lesbian, Gay, Bisexual and Transgender Youth," *Journal of Adolescent Health* 59, no. 6 (July 2016): 674–80, accessed June 1, 2019, https://www.ncbi.nlm.nih.gov/pubmed/27707515.

28 Kristina R. Olson, Lily Durwood, Madeleine DeMeules, and Katie A. McLaughlin. "Mental Health of Transgender Children Who Are Supported in Their Identities," *Pediatrics* 137, no. 3 (March 2016), accessed June 1, 2019, https://pediatrics.aappublications.org/content/137/3/e20153223.

29 Stephen T. Russell, Amanda M. Pollitt, Gu Li, and Arnold H. Grossman, "Chosen Name Use Is Linked to Reduced Depressive Symptoms, Suicidal Ideation, and Suicidal Behavior among Transgender Youth," *Journal of Adolescent Health* 63,

no. 4 (March 2018): 501–5, accessed June 1, 2019, https://www.ncbi.nlm.nih.gov/pubmed/29609917.

30 Ilan H. Meyer, Feijun Luo, Bianca D.M. Wilson, and Deborah M. Stone, "Sexual Orientation Enumeration in State Antibullying Statutes in the United States: Associations with Bullying, Suicidal Ideation, and Suicide Attempts Among Youth," *LGBT Health* 6, no. 1 (January 2019): 9–14, accessed June 1, 2019, https://www.ncbi.nlm.nih.gov/pubmed/30638436.

2

Informed Consent for Intersex Children

Katharine B. Dalke

In the summer of 2018, I found myself observing a protest on the front steps of a children's hospital. Activists of diverse genders, ages, colors, and abilities wearing identical bright yellow tee shirts had come together from all over the country—and from across the world. Sharing a megaphone, protestors told the supportive crowd their stories of having intersex identities and bodies, bodies that had been concealed and, in some cases, irrevocably altered, by well-intentioned physicians and surgeons. Varying as the narratives were, they were unified by experiences of medically sanctioned, traumatic loss of autonomy in the pursuit of normalcy, a legacy of physical and emotional pain, and, above all, a call for health care professionals to listen, learn, and change their practices.

It is on these stories that this chapter is centered. Informed consent and shared decision-making are essential to the provision of quality care for people with intersex conditions. I would know. I'm one of these people.

I was the firstborn child of parents who had fallen in love in their first semester of medical school. Although the first six years of my life were full, with the arrival of my siblings, fraternal twins, and my parents' medical training, nothing was out of the ordinary. At age six, I underwent a routine hernia operation. My surgeon and parents were shocked to discover that in place of ovaries and a uterus, my pelvis carried internal testes. A karyotype confirmed that my sex chromosomes were XY, instead of the typical female XX. My diagnosis, which would later be known as Complete Androgen Insensitivity Syndrome, reflected my body's inability to respond to the androgens that my testes had produced during fetal development, shifting me instead down a "usual" female pathway.

The next ten years were excruciating for me and my family. My physician, a well-respected pediatric endocrinologist, followed a then standard medical practice, recommending that my parents never disclose to me my diagnosis, chromosomes, or gonads. Intersex patients who knew, they feared, would question their gender identity and sexual orientation or commit suicide. And so my family adhered diligently to the prescription of total secrecy, each of us internalizing the message that there was something wrong or shameful about my natural body. It wasn't until we found the Androgen Insensitivity Syndrome-Differences of Sex Development Support Group that my family could begin to visualize a future in which I knew all the details of my condition, and I was loved and happy for being different.

Since my first support group meeting, when I was seventeen years old, I have met hundreds of intersex youth and adults and parents of intersex youth. Just as every other aspect of our identities varies, so too do our specific intersex conditions and experiences. Some of us have typical genitals, and others have larger than average clitorises, smaller than usual penises, or genitalia that do not immediately resemble either; some of us had genital surgery in infancy, adolescence, adulthood, or not at all; some of us are overall at peace with our medical care, and many of us are enraged. We identify as queer or intersex or having an intersex condition or a difference of sex development. Regardless of our differences, we all intersect at a shared experience of bodies that do not align with typical definitions of male or female and understand the accompanying shame, stigma, and isolation. We also understand that loving and accepting our bodies is an act of radical resistance.

Historically, we intersex people have been seen as an "experiment of nature"—variations that at once illustrate "normal" sex development and threaten the cis and heteronormative orders.[1] One of medicine's roles throughout history has been to serve as a means of correcting what is deemed by the society to be abnormal, and we are a particularly striking example of this.

Starting in the 1950s, gender identity was theorized to be determined by nurture rather than nature, and as such could be "assigned."[2] This supposition was hugely appealing to providers and families faced with the "social emergency" of a child with obvious genital difference, whose biological sex and therefore gender were not readily discerned. In response, physicians, surgeons, and psychologists recommended surgical "correction" of genitals—usually informed by surgical capability and future capacity for penetrative heterosexual intercourse—even in cases in which the child's immediate medical health was not in any way affected by their genitals. To ensure the best outcome, which was defined by a lack of ambiguity in gender identity, role, or sexual orientation, all diagnostic information was concealed, including from many parents. Irreversible surgical interventions were performed in infancy or toddlerhood. As a result, virtually all young patients and many of their caregivers were denied the opportunity to give informed consent.

Even people with typical genitals and those who did not have surgery were still subject to loss of decision-making autonomy. Lack of diagnostic information meant that even if a person participated in a decision about their medical care, they usually did not understand the reasons for the care. Some people report that their doctors outright lied to them to explain a need for a medication, exam, or procedure in adolescence or adulthood. Additionally, many people participated in unnecessary, intrusive, and objectifying physical examination and medical photography without consent, with some finding photographs of themselves published in scientific journals and books.[3]

In the 1990s, the intersex advocacy movement was born, under the umbrella of the Intersex Society of North America, which highlighted the physical and psychological harm that many people suffered under this model of care. Activists bravely revealed the shame, stigma, isolation, loss of sexual sensation, genital pain, urinary incontinence, and multiple recurrent surgeries that they experienced as a result of procedures they never consented to.

At the same time, the gender theory that had undergirded the model was debunked, and physicians and surgeons began to critically reevaluate best practices.[4] A landmark, if incomplete, Consensus Statement was published in 2006, recommending disclosure of diagnoses, more conservative surgical management, and treatment in interdisciplinary teams, which allows for more thoughtful and evidence-based decision-making.[5]

Today, a growing number of families are choosing deferral of medically unnecessary surgeries, a stance which has been supported by multiple human rights groups and medical organizations, including United

Nations experts on health, torture, and women's and children's rights, Human Rights Watch, Physicians for Human Rights, the American Academy of Family Physicians, and GLMA: Health Professionals for LGBTQ Equality.[6] These positions are grounded in the recognition that people, especially children, have a human right to bodily autonomy, an open future, and informed consent. Nevertheless, early, irreversible, and elective interventions are still recommended and performed throughout the United States, and many intersex adults continue to recover from the traumatic medical interventions and encounters they have experienced.[7]

In addition to the ethical and legal concerns applicable to all patient care, ensuring informed consent in the process of delivering care to intersex people is an essential and reparative step that addresses the harm inflicted upon intersex people. Explicit informed consent, including the rationale, benefits, and risks should be obtained for even apparently straightforward procedures for patients; these might include physical exams, inclusion of nonessential staff or health professions learners in examinations, medical photography, and non-intersex-related health care.

Informed consent must be especially intentional and thorough when discussing irreversible interventions with families of children. In these cases, families must understand the substantial risks of surgery, including sexual and urinary dysfunction and the need for surgical revisions. When gender is surgically assigned, it can severely exacerbate the symptoms of and limit medical affirmation options for gender dysphoria later in life. Both community narratives and a growing evidence base show that the incidence of transgender and nonbinary identities are substantially higher than in the general population for some groups of intersex people. These risks must be balanced against the putative benefits of surgery. Cited benefits tend to include normalizing the appearance of the genitals, reducing psychosocial distress, and promoting psychosocial health, which, as three former U.S. surgeon generals wrote, have not actually been proven.[8]

Providers must also be mindful that there are many barriers to obtaining effective informed consent. In the case of surgical decision-making regarding an infant with atypical genitals, parents are often uncertain about the implications of their child's condition, which may engender anxiety and urgency and impact decision-making. Because intersex conditions are relatively rare and heterogeneous, there is often a lack of robust evidence available to guide providers and families in anticipating outcomes. Adolescents, especially those with intersecting vulnerable identities, may struggle with trust and engagement with the team due to previous non-affirming or even discriminatory experiences. Finally, personal and societal bias and stigma against nonnormative bodies can be heightened and exacerbated by the stress of making a decision in what can feel like a vacuum. Helping families and youth visualize a positive future with a nonnormative body is critical for addressing bias, and role models from support groups can be life-changing.

Fortunately, excellent work has been done to promote best practices in the care of intersex youth and adults.[9] Families and doctors should be encouraged to disclose information to children and to defer any irreversible and elective intervention until children are able to meaningfully participate in the decision. LGBT-inclusive providers will recognize that these practices are affirming, grounded in collaborative decision-making over a longitudinal relationship with reflexive acceptance of patients' bodies and identities. Encouraging youth to explore their identities and sexualities and how their bodies align with these can help youth and providers feel more confident in the decisions they make. Specific practices are trauma-informed, recognizing that it is incumbent on providers to build trust and engagement, which can be accomplished through minimization of unnecessary exams, clear explanations of procedures, and use of inclusive and affirming language. LGBT providers, however, must also be mindful that many intersex people identify as heterosexual and/or have a cisgender experience, and no assumptions should be made about any patient's identity or comfort in queer spaces.

During that protest last summer, I declined the megaphone, preferring instead to listen and learn from people I love and people I didn't yet know. Had I spoken, I would have shouted a message to a younger me and the younger selves of my parents and doctors: "This body is beautiful, and this person is stronger and smarter than you assume. Teach me about my body, and I'll teach you about myself. We can figure this out together."

Katharine Dalke, MD, MBE, is an assistant professor of psychiatry at Penn State and attending psychiatrist at Pennsylvania Psychiatric Institute, with clinical and academic expertise in the psychiatric care and support of patients with diverse experiences of sex, gender, and sexuality. Dr. Dalke has been appointed to the Pennsylvania Commission on LGBTQ Affairs and the Transgender Working Group at the Pennsylvania Department of Health and has been recognized by the community with advocacy awards. She also serves as the director of the Office for Culturally Responsive Education at the Penn State College of Medicine, focusing on training health care professionals to provide excellent, intersectionally aware health care to patients of diverse backgrounds. Dr. Dalke is a graduate of Haverford College and the University of Pennsylvania School of Medicine, from which she also earned a Masters in Bioethics, completing her psychiatry residency at the Hospital of the University of Pennsylvania.

Notes

1 Alice Domurat Dreger, *Hermaphrodites and the Medical Invention of Sex* (Cambridge, MA: Harvard University Press, 1998).

2 Joanne Money, Joan G. Hampson, and John L. Hampson, "Hermaphroditism: Recommendations Concerning Assignment of Sex, Change of Sex, and Psychologic Management," *Bulletin of Johns Hopkins Hospital* 97, no. 4 (October 1955): 284–300.

3 Milton Diamond, "Sex, Gender, and Identity Over the Years: A Changing Perspective," *Child and Adolescent Psychiatric Clinics of North America* 13, no. 3 (July 2004): 591–607, accessed June 1, 2019, https://www.childpsych.theclinics.com/article/S1056-4993(04)00010-0/abstract.

4 M. Diamond and H.K. Sigmundson, "Sex Reassignment at Birth: Long-Term Review and Clinical Implications," *Archives of Pediatric and Adolescent Medicine* 151, no. 3 (March 1997): 298–304, accessed June 1, 2019, http://www.hawaii.edu/PCSS/biblio/articles/1961to1999/1997-sex-reassignment.html.

5 Peter A. Lee, Christopher P. Houk, S. Faisal Ahmed, Ieuan A. Hughes, with the International Consensus Conference on Intersex, "Consensus Statement on Management of Intersex Disorders," *Pediatrics* 118, no. 2 (August 2006): 488–500, accessed June 1, 2019, https://bit.ly/2QAbAle.

6 "Research & Policy Statements Supporting Intersex Bodily Autonomy & Improved Care," *interACT*, accessed June 1, 2019, https://interactadvocates.org/intersex-medical-policy-and-research/#statements.

7 Human Rights Watch and interact, *"I Want To Be Like Nature Made Me": Medically Unnecessary Surgeries on Children in the US* (New York: Human Rights Watch, 2017), accessed June 1, 2019, https://www.hrw.org/sites/default/files/report_pdf/lgbtintersex0717_web_0.pdf.

8 M. Joycelyn Elders, David Satcher, and Richard Carmona, "Re-Thinking Genital Surgeries on Intersex Infants," Palm Center: Blueprints for Sound Public Policy, June 2017, accessed June 1, 2019, www.palmcenter.org/wp-content/uploads/2017/06/Re-Thinking-Genital-Surgeries-1.pdf.

9 interact and Lambda Legal, *Providing Ethical and Compassionate Health Care to Intersex Patients: Intersex-Affirming Hospital Policies*, July 2018, accessed June 1, 2019, https://www.lambdalegal.org/sites/default/files/publications/downloads/resource_20180731_hospital-policies-intersex.pdf.

3

Navigating Pediatric Care for Transgender Youth

Alisa Bowman

When I learned that my second grader was transgender, I found myself explaining who my child was—over and over again—to a long list of people: my parents, my husband's parents, my siblings, extended family, teachers, administrators, friends, parents of my child's friends; it went on and on.

One person I didn't bother to tell: my child's pediatrician.

I ghosted him instead.

At the time, I didn't even know why. I'd never heard anyone in that particular doctor's office say anything offensive. Yet, I just couldn't shake the feeling that my son's first doctor would either be completely uninformed (best-case scenario) or openly hostile (worst-case scenario). Now, years later, with the benefit of hindsight, I know precisely what made me uneasy. It had nothing to do with what my son's doctor said or did. Rather, it had everything to do with what he did not say or do: talk to us about our child's gender.

My transgender son had never behaved, presented himself, or carried himself like a typical girl. By second grade, his short hair was nearly buzzed and he wore ties and only allowed me to shop for him in the boy's section of the department store. His hobbies centered on watching World Wrestling Entertainment, memorizing Pokémon characters, and playing Bakugan and kickball. His transness was on full display—and loudly noticeable to just about anyone who had the slightest inkling of the science of gender diversity.

During several doctor's visits, I'd even mentioned telling signs—how my child refused to go to the bathroom at school, for example. There had been plenty of openings. Yet our pediatrician never once asked us questions about our son's gender nor suggested that our child might be trans. It was akin to treating a child with high blood sugar and never once saying anything to the child's parents about type 1 diabetes.

I also knew that this doctor was extremely religious, and one election season he'd plastered his waiting room with Republican signs. Sure, there are plenty of pro-equality religious people as well as pro-equality Republicans. But some of the loudest anti-trans narratives come from the religious right. Because of that, these two details made me uneasy.

So I ghosted him. I just stopped making well visit appointments.

Instead, for my son's medical care, I began traveling well over an hour to Philadelphia and an LGBT clinic where a transgender provider had a growing practice that included dozens and dozens of trans youth.

As soon as I walked into the clinic, I knew we were home. Pro-equality stickers and messages decorated the office. Intake forms asked about our child's pronouns and chosen name and not a single person misgendered him. A social worker interviewed us thoroughly, gently, and confidently, asking a series of questions that my son's previous doctor had either been too embarrassed, too inept, or too dismissive to broach. The whole atmosphere felt warm, safe, inviting, and comfortable. At our former provider, my son had been mostly shy and silent, answering his doctor's questions quietly, with only a few words. But now, with his new provider, he bloomed. He chatted comfortably and easily with his new doctor and began participating in his care with a new level of interest. We were in good hands.

My husband and I both work full-time, so you can probably imagine our difficulty in getting our son to a doctor who was so far away. Here's why we stayed with this clinic for years.

The clinic's primary health care provider was one of the top experts in the country. I found it deeply comforting that our new provider not only cared for dozens of transgender children but also regularly attended gender conferences, and even served as a mentor to other doctors who were learning how to care for trans youth.

The clinic was a completely safe space. It was clear to me that the front office staff were not only highly trained at getting names and pronouns correct, they were also trained in warmth and understanding. The office itself was highly secure, and our privacy was always respected.

The clinic put wellness ahead of profits. At the time, insurance often didn't cover trans care. When insurance did cover it, high deductibles, steep co-pays, and out-of-pocket caps often made care cost prohibitive. The clinic used a sliding scale when it billed, and every request for money came with a question, "Is that okay?" It was clear to me that every single person who worked at the clinic cared more about my son getting the medicine and tests that he needed than they cared about my ability to pay for it all.

In particular, the medicines used to stop puberty in trans youth can cost well over thirty thousand dollars a year. Even with a drug plan that covers 80 percent, a family is looking at a six thousand–dollar yearly pharmacy bill—and that's often in addition to a more than three thousand–dollar deductible. For working-class people, these prices are completely out of reach.

I showed up to one visit in tears after a pharmacy had sent me an eleven thousand–dollar bill that I had not been expecting and had no idea how I would pay. My entire body was shaking as I told my son's doctor, "I don't know how I'm going to keep my son on these medicines for several more years. I don't know what to do. How do people do this?" My son's doctor wrapped his hands around mine and said, "Alisa, we can help you." And he and his staff filled out the paperwork needed for my son to receive these medicines at a much reduced price.

The clinic treated the whole child and even the whole family. In addition to well visits for our child, the clinic offered a support group for parents of transgender children, offered free legal clinics, organized a free yearly conference, and even organized fun outings to skating rinks and other locations.

Our health care provider had a list of other gender affirming health care providers. This made it so much easier and faster to find specialists, counselors, and more.

The clinic did everything they could to make health care possible. Our son's doctor often called us to go over our medical questions rather than have us travel to Philadelphia to have the same conversation. He also shifted his schedule several times to accommodate ours—even once coming in on his day off, because it was the only day I could get my child to the city. Such acts would no doubt be appreciated by anyone in need of health care, but I found them especially helpful, given that my son not only saw his primary care doctor several times a year but also saw an endocrinologist every six months and regularly needed blood work and other testing.

The clinic hired people who looked like my son. Gender-diverse people worked in the front office, as nurses and phlebotomists, and even as my son's primary care provider.

Not long ago, my son's provider left the clinic for a new position at a different facility. It was only then that I considered finding a primary care provider closer to home. I'd heard of an affirming doctor with a practice mere minutes from my house. I'd been told that she too saw dozens of transgender patients. I decided to check her out.

When we walked in, I couldn't help but notice a rainbow sticker near the check-in area. The forms asked about chosen names and pronouns, and everything about the office felt warm and friendly. As a gender-expansive nurse took my son's vitals, I was pretty sure I'd found our new home—and I was right.

Alisa Bowman is a professional writer, editor, and marketer who works for one of the world's largest media companies. Along with Michele Angello, she's the co-author of *Raising the Transgender Child*. She moderates a support group for parents of transgender children, advocates for trans youth and their families, and is the parent of an incredible boy, who just so happens to be trans.

4

Not Your Average Sex Talk

Emmett Patterson

> When an adult teaches young people, the message is heard as a whisper. When a peer educator teaches, it is heard as a shout.
>
> —Dr. Mary Jo Podgurski

I fear for the person who types anything into my computer's search bar. What they find won't be pretty: questions about alternatives to anal beads, symptoms of gonorrhea, if sex toys can get through customs in Peru. As much as my own sex life is exciting, it isn't *pages and pages of blush-worthy Google searches* exciting. But when you're a queer sex educator, you tend to search for answers to questions that others might not want to ask, haven't thought to ask, and, often, questions that don't have clear answers.

Questions create the foundation of what we do not yet know; asking the right ones can help us learn about anything and everything, including about people who are rendered invisible in the quest to get those answers. For LGBT people, this invisibility prevents us from knowing quite a bit about our lives, particularly about our sexual health. It is not for lack of interest or trying that we find ourselves struggling to answer our most simple and vital questions about our bodies. The sex education system in this country is broken for all young people, but LGBT young people feel this brokenness even more intensely. We navigate an educational system that lacks clarity on specific, medically accurate, and affirming sexual health information for us as queer people. Due to a complicated history of federal funding that often pits religious values against science, LGBT-exclusionary sex education has been the norm in the United States.

The situation is bleak for LGBT young people who are excluded from even the most comprehensive curriculum, which often centers around pregnancy prevention and does not address the kinds of health concerns specific to LGBT people. In other words, existing sex education curricula do not simply ignore LGBT young people; they outright demonize them. No matter where we go, what kind of community we visit, or the current political climate of our country, an overwhelming majority of the young activists we meet share that they are disappointed and, in fact, outraged with the sex education they received growing up. And when you look at the research, there's no arguing against their outrage. According to the Guttmacher Institute, twenty-four states and the District of Columbia mandate sex education.[1] Only twelve states require discussion of sexual orientation in the curriculum, with nine states requiring discussion of sexual orientation be inclusive and three states including only negative information on sexual orientation.[2] From start to finish, of the fifty United States and DC, only nine jurisdictions include positive information on LGBT-related content in schools.[3] Additionally, only 8 percent to 44 percent of schools actually provided LGBT-inclusive sex education, demonstrating that the majority of states permitting the inclusion of LGBT topics did not end up including them in their curriculum.[4]

This reality sets up young LGBT people to experience negative sexual health outcomes as they move through the world as adolescents and into adulthood. For example, exclusionary sex education heightens the minority stress factors that impact us as LGBT people, worsening existing health disparities that result from interpersonal discrimination and structural violence.[5] Lesbian, gay, and bisexual cisgender teenagers are twice as likely to experience unplanned pregnancy as their straight peers.[6] For young gay and bisexual cisgender men, HIV rates continue to increase; gay and bisexual men of color face the burden of HIV diagnoses: one in four Latino gay and bisexual men and one in two Black gay and bisexual men will be diagnosed with HIV in their lifetime.[7] Information about bisexual people is often only available within aggregate data of gay and lesbian respondents, making it difficult to assess specific sexual health issues impacting bisexual people.[8] Finally, as with many health issues, research rarely documents the needs of trans, nonbinary, and gender nonconforming young people, but what we do know is that transgender women of color experience the worldwide burden of HIV, and more than 95 percent of transgender men report knowing nothing about their sexual health needs.[9] In other words, LGBT young people face a burden of negative health outcomes related to sex and intimacy, including an epidemic of intimate partner violence,[10] having sex while intoxicated,[11] and being unable to access preventive health care and relevant sexual health information.[12]

So, yes, LGBT young people are enraged and rightfully so.

•

I know what it feels like when curricula and medical institutions are not structured around your sexual and gender-related needs; these experiences built my consciousness around health inequalities and pushed me to develop my own skills as an educator and activist. As a young person living in a rural community outside of Pittsburgh, Pennsylvania, coming out as a trans man to my family and community brought a number of challenges to my sexual health. In my mandated year of psychotherapy that I completed to receive approval for hormone therapy and other transition-related care, countless providers ignored discussing my sexual and reproductive health. The first time I was asked if I had thought about becoming pregnant in the future was right after my primary care physician placed my first hormone shot in my hands. My providers seemed to not be bothered to think about or, perhaps, couldn't imagine a trans person being sexual, which prevented them from assessing what some of my sexual health concerns might be. So I stayed silent and researched on my own, struggling to find myself in news stories about teen pregnancy and deciphering if HPV vaccine guidelines applied to trans men.

During my first years living as a college student in Washington, DC, my concerns about my sexual health became more urgent. A doctor at a local DC hospital gave me a forced pelvic exam in front of medical students when I had come into the emergency room after a possible concussion. After that, I suffered from abdominal cramping and random pelvic bleeding. I tried and failed to navigate sex with cisgender queer men but stopped using condoms when these sexual partners told me no one else would sleep with me if I used them. While on hormones, I became pregnant and had a miscarriage less than two months in. The powerlessness I felt to make informed decisions about my body turned into rage. It built and built until it had nowhere else to go.

In November 2013, that rage turned into action. My dear friend Lex Loro and I were students together at American University, walking into our first event as part of the campus queer student group. We expanded the existing queer women's sex talk to be a queer sex talk inclusive of all sexual orientations, gender identities, and expressions. We called the event Not Your Average Sex Talk, which would later become the name of our organization focused on training young queer and trans activists to create their own sex education events in their communities. Prior to meeting in DC, both Lex and I worked to expand sexual health information to include LGBT young people in our respective communities. We wanted to continue supporting sex education efforts rooted in relevant, affirming information about queer health, bodies, and identities. Queer sexual liberation fueled our activism, and part of that liberation called for openly discussing how we intimately connect with each other.

The conference room filled with chattering first-years and prematurely gray-haired juniors stifling their panic as mid-term deadlines loomed. The event start time grew closer and closer. The sex educator from a local queer health clinic still had not arrived. We called them, but their phone rang and rang. We and the nearly seventy students who had packed themselves into the conference room waited. Fifteen minutes after our event was supposed to begin, Lex and I accepted the fact that the educator was not coming. It was not the first time in my life—and in the lives of many in the room—that an adult failed to show up. Lex and I looked at each other, sharing one of those perfect telepathic moments that queer people sometimes share. Both of us had been instrumental in transforming the sex education in our conservative small towns. As queer people, we had plenty of sexy, horrific, and empowering stories to share. Who was to say *we* couldn't lead the discussion? In a room packed with our fellow anxious and eager students, Lex whispered in my ear, "Can we do this ourselves?"

We asked everyone to rearrange the chairs from classroom style to a circle. From the very beginning, we wanted our fellow students to feel that they could share and teach as much as they could absorb and learn. We opened the conversation by specifying that we are not medical providers or licensed counselors but concerned young queer people who wanted to do better by our community. Our role that evening would be to hear from queer people about what they did and did not know about their bodies and have them share their experiences of erasure in sex education.

That evening, Lex and I began uncovering answers to some of the questions regarding queer health thereby laying the foundation for a new way to talk about sexual health and wellness with our peers. What we found in the first of our many sex talks was that something incredible happened when young people led the conversation: others around them authentically opened up, shared deeper, reached into themselves to pull out their most trying concerns more than we had ever seen when adult facilitators led the discussion. Some students in our circle shared that the sex education they received in school only discussed gay men in conversations about HIV. Others chimed in, saying they had only heard about condoms and pregnancy prevention. Even more shuddered in horror, flashing back to the frightening images of chlamydia and gonorrhea that their health teachers projected on the white board. Others in the room felt offended by their inadequate, abstinence-only sex education or by not having received any at all. Sexual health and wellness for all of us, but especially queer people, goes beyond condom demonstrations and cringe inducing pictures of STIs. In the room on that November night, our people rallied around each other proving just that, by discussing consent, desexualization as a result of their body size, navigating sexual racism, and asking about how to have great anal sex.

In just two hours, we began breaking down the barriers that so many of us felt from the adults in our life who tried to teach us about sex and failed. We didn't want to be talked down to; rather, we wanted the space to air our concerns and work with our friends and peers to create realistic strategies that made us feel control over our bodies, often for the first time in our lives. We realized we were giving the sex talk we had needed all along.

•

Are there condoms for tongues? Can vegans be in the leather community? What do you do when you fart in someone's mouth while they're eating your ass?

After years of working in sexual health, I have become adept at answering hilarious questions, ones that seem to get less and less hypothetical with every sex talk I facilitate. In our time supporting young people through Not Your Average Sex Talk, we have found that laughter is often the uniting force within our work. The rigidity of traditional sex education, with its reliance on scare tactics, colors sex as an experience that is gravely serious and, particularly for queer people, dangerous. When young people first walk into the room where we will facilitate the discussion, they often are looking down or folding into themselves, apparently triggered by memories of high school sex education classes: gym teachers yelling at them to use condoms, spiritual leaders screaming until blue in the face, "Wait!"—generation upon generation of adults who were never taught to embrace their sexuality failing to prepare young people to embrace theirs. As peer facilitators, we had a matter of minutes to unravel years of shame and embarrassment around queer sex so that young people could be fully present.

Humor is one of our most effective tools in doing that. In Not Your Average Sex Talk, we allow participants to periodically submit their questions anonymously, either online before the event or during the discussion on note cards. What queer people ask ranges from the heartbreaking to the thoughtful to the hilarious. Questions that make the room erupt in laughter—or turn even my face beet red—time and time again reinforce my belief in the resilience of young people. Finding the humor in queer sex is challenging. The horrors experienced in the AIDS epidemic anchor our collective history as queer people living in the U.S. The resulting fears from that time still emanate throughout our communities, particularly stigma against people living with HIV. We were told for so long that our queer bodies were inherently dangerous and not worthy of love or pleasure that eventually we all believed it. Some of us still do.

•

I was raped a few months ago. Will anyone ever want to have sex with me again?

Other questions young LGBT people ask us often challenge us to address trauma. We consistently hear from queer survivors of sexual assault. What they bring into the space in their vulnerability is important for everyone in that room to hear: their fears around connecting with other people, what this means for their sex life, and gut-wrenching questioning of their worth as a person. Affirmations inherent in the answers to these kinds of questions are important for every young queer person to hear, not just survivors of assault.

I stare at this particular question, quickly scrawled over the crumpled pink index card I held in my hands. Taking a pause, I looked up. The faces in the room stared back, some showing immediate recognition of themselves in that question.

Only a week before, I opened my bleary eyes in the middle of the night, finding myself draped on top of my bed, fully clothed and disoriented. Immediately, something felt off. Lifting myself from the bed, I staggered out of my bedroom and into the adjacent living room. My front door, open wide, led to a chilly December night. Fallen leaves swirled into my apartment, collecting at my feet. I ran to the bathroom and vomited. I woke up there a few hours later. I stripped off my clothes and slowly began to realize someone had raped me. Having no memory of what happened, I realized someone had drugged me to do it.

Fresh in my mind, I brought myself back to the group. I inhaled, deep. All of the air inside of me shot out in a forceful sigh. This question, which previously had not hit quite so close to home, now sounded strangely familiar, echoing my own recent fears of future intimacy.

Tears welled up in my eyes, and I uttered, "I'm afraid of that, too."

The barriers innate in traditional sex education spaces came crashing down. Tearfully opening up about my own history of assault connected me to everyone in that room, not just the survivor.

When we take on the teacher role, we often forget the experiences that drive us to do this work. I certainly did. This moment, and each moment of vulnerability Lex and I share as facilitators, transform our fears, anxieties, and uncertainties into powerful teaching tools. These allow all of us to breathe a sigh of relief and feel a little less isolated. We reveal those difficult experiences to others, like leaves rushing through the door piling at our feet, letting the outside world come in for just a little while.

•

Why do I feel so guilty after having sex?

The chance to learn about sexual and gender identity exploration is at the core of LGBT exclusion in sex education curricula. My straight peers didn't need someone to walk them through coming to terms with being straight or cisgender. Those are the defaults in life and in sex education. But how different would my coming to terms with being queer and trans have been if I had been told people like me even existed?

This gap necessitates affirmation being core to our work through Not Your Average Sex Talk. Our very presence as queer people in a leadership role demonstrates that all of us are worthy of taking up space, and that we are experts on our own people. Affirmation is terribly sought after through questions begging for assurance that all of the violence is not a result of them being abnormal but a result of hate from the world wherein we live. Questions like, *Is this okay? Am I normal? How do I do this?* keep me up at night. They are the same questions I have asked myself countless times. Talking about sexual and gender identity in our sex talks cannot answer the unanswerable, but it certainly makes young people feel real in a world that renders them invisible, especially for those who have multiple marginalized identities as queer and trans people of color and disabled people.

We affirm the identities of youth activists beyond their queerness. Lex and I don't often hit the road to convene people like we did at the start; rather, we now commit ourselves to support the professional development of young queer sexual health activists. As Not Your Average Sex Talk transformed from a pop-up sex education program into an activist training network, we realized our power to affirm young queer people as leaders completely capable of transforming their communities, just like we were. In this new chapter, we partner with young leaders and the organizations that support them to improve sexual health and wellness in their communities. We provide technical assistance, training, and coaching to young sex educators across the U.S., tailored to their individual needs. With our help, young people are creating safer spaces to talk about queer sex and intimacy. We are helping them develop critical skills, like group facilitation, responding to trauma, and building cross-movement partnerships.

My absolute payout in this work is the stories activists tell us about their own not so average sex talks; from a dinner party discussion of Black trans men navigating sex, race, and disability to university students in the South organizing against LGBT sexual violence on their campus to asexual women cultivating new practices of intimacy, we find the spirit of Not Your Average Sex Talk everywhere. Because at the end of the day, those questions that drip with the fear of not belonging do have answers: *You are okay. You are normal. Do it your own way.*

•

Questions hold the power to form the foundation of what we do not yet know. Their power does not make them any less scary; I am still afraid that we will always have more questions than answers in this volatile time to be young and LGBT. With sex education curricula relentlessly under attack, pressured to be centered around abstinence solely, and, even in the most comprehensive curriculum, continuing to exclusively focus on the needs of straight, cisgender young people, I believe we have plenty more work to do to make sex education realistic, inclusive, and accessible for all young people who need it.

Not Your Average Sex Talk cannot change the medical realities for young queer and trans people when it comes to their sexual health. Neither can we connect every young person living with HIV to treatment nor can we eliminate the hate that queer and trans people face in their communities. No matter how many stories we tell, we cannot support every survivor of sexual assault that struggles to connect with new partners. But with every young person we support, we can rest assured knowing we are creating a movement of leaders who can.

Emmett Patterson is a queer health activist, a writer, and The Global Health Projects Manager at Grindr for Equality. He studied Public Health and Women's, Gender, and Sexuality Studies at American University and completed a graduate certificate in LGBT Health Policy and Practice at George Washington University. His work focuses on transmasculine sexual health and trauma. He is the cofounder of Not Your Average Sex Talk, a peer-to-peer sex education activist training program that prepares young queer and trans activists to create their own spaces for sexual health and wellness programming. At Grindr, he oversees health programs, projects, and campaigns for LGBT users worldwide.

Notes

1 "Sex and HIV Education," Guttmacher Institute, May 1, 2019, accessed June 1, 2019, https://www.guttmacher.org/state-policy/explore/sex-and-hiv-education.

2 Ibid.

3 Advocates for Youth, Answer, GLSEN, Human Rights Campaign (HRC) Foundation, Planned Parenthood Federation of America (PPFA), and Sexuality Information and Education Council of the United States (SIECUS), "A Call to Action: LGBTQ Youth Need Inclusive Sex Education," Human Rights Campaign, 2015, accessed June 1, 2019, https://www.hrc.org/resources/a-call-to-action-lgbtq-youth-need-inclusive-sex-education.

4 Zewditu Demissie, Nancy D. Brener, Tim McManus, Shari L. Shanklin, Joseph Hawkins, and Laura Kann, *School Health Profiles 2014: Characteristics of Health Programs among Secondary Schools* (Washington, DC: United States Department of Health and Human Services, Centers for Disease Control and Prevention, 2015), accessed June 1, 2019, www.cdc.gov/healthyyouth/data/profiles/pdf/2014/2014_Profiles_Report.pdf.

5 Advocates for Youth et al., "A Call to Action."

6 Andrew M. Seaman, "Pregnancies More Common among Lesbian, Gay, Bisexual Youths," Reuters, May 14, 2015, accessed June 1, 2019, https://www.reuters.com/article/us-pregnancy-teen-lgbt/pregnancies-more-common-among-lesbian-gay-bisexual-youths-idUSKBN0NZ2AT20150514.

7 United States Department of Health and Human Services, "Half of Black Gay Men and a Quarter of Latino Gay Men Projected to Be Diagnosed within Their Lifetime" (press release), Centers for Disease Control and Prevention, February 23, 2016, accessed June 1, 2019, https://www.cdc.gov/nchhstp/newsroom/2016/croi-press-release-risk.html.

8 Shabab Ahmed Mirza, "Disaggregating the Data for Bisexual People," Center for American Progress, September 24, 2018, accessed June 1, 2019, https://www.americanprogress.org/issues/lgbt/reports/2018/09/24/458472/disaggregating-data-bisexual-people/.

9 Stefan D. Baral, Tonia Poteat, Susanne Strömdahl, Andrea L. Wirtz, Thomas E. Guadamuz, and Chris Beyrer, "Worldwide Burden of HIV in Transgender Women: A Systematic Review and Meta-Analysis," *Lancet Infectious Diseases* 13, no. 3 (December 2012): 214–22, accessed June 1, 2019, www.thelancet.com/journals/laninf/article/PIIS1473-3099(12)70315-8/fulltext; Jaime M. Grant, Lisa A. Mottet, and Justin Tanis, with Jack Harrison-Quintana, Jody L. Herman, and Mara Keisling, *Injustice at Every Turn: A Report of the National Transgender Discrimination Survey* (Washington, DC: National Center for Transgender Equity/National Gay and Lesbian Taskforce, 2011), accessed June 1, 2019, https://transequality.org/sites/default/files/docs/resources/NTDS_Report.pdf.

10 T.R. Reuter, M.E. Newcomb, S.W. Whitton, and B. Mustanski, "Intimate Partner Violence Victimization in LGBT Young Adults: Demographic Differences and Associations with Health Behaviors," *Psychology of Violence* 7, no. 1 (January 2017): 1–9, accessed June 1, 2019, https://www.ncbi.nlm.nih.gov/pubmed/28451465.

11 A.L. Herrick, M.P. Marshal, H.A. Smith, G. Sucato, and R.D. Stall, "Sex While Intoxicated: A Meta-Analysis Comparing Heterosexual and Sexual Minority Youth," *Journal of Adolescent Health* 48, no. 3 (March 2011): 306–9, accessed June 1, 2019, https://www.ncbi.nlm.nih.gov/pubmed/21338904.

12 "GLSEN Calls for LGBTQ-Inclusive Sex Ed" (press release), GLSEN, December 2, 2015, accessed June 1, 2019, https://www.glsen.org/article/lack-comprehensive-sex-education-putting-lgbtq-youth-risk-national-organizations-issue-call.

5

Resiliency for Homeless Queer Youth

Arin Jayes

LGBT youth are interesting, curious, passionate, and self-motivated. They strive for independence and take risks. However, they experience unique challenges in figuring out who they are and who they are attracted to in a society that does not understand them. The discrimination that LGBT youth face places them at high risk for becoming victims of discrimination, verbal harassment, and physical violence.[1] All too often they are left to face formidable obstacles alone, without the external supports that foster both safety and healthy development. On top of that, most youth are legally and financially dependent on adults, and when parents find queer sexualities and gender nonconformity to be unfamiliar territory, they find themselves unsure of how to respond.[2] Thus, many LGBT youth maintain resilience by relying on each other's support—whether it is through peer support groups, reaching out to each other on the internet, or forming community coalitions.

Like many queer and trans people, I wanted to effect positive change for queer youth, because I can remember how important that support is. I am queer and trans identified, privileged by family support, access to higher education, and my race. Yet even with my social privileges, I remember what it's like to be a queer youth, and how important it is to teach strategies of resiliency to populations who need them most. I wanted to answer the question: What types of enrichment programs help LGBT youth build resilience and leadership in their communities?

In response to this question, I partnered with Casa Ruby, an LGBT homeless shelter in Washington, DC, to work with their youth program participants to create a youth-written and operated blog. The photos, essays, videos, poems, visual art, and short stories on the blog focused on the experience of being a homeless LGBT youth in DC and the tools of resilience that the youth use to combat homophobia, transphobia, and racism in their daily lives. The goal was to empower homeless LGBT youth to be leaders in their community and to be their own self-advocates. Through sharing their life experiences, they could build resilience in the face of oppression and ultimately affect local and national public policy.

The concept of resilience grew out of the discipline of developmental psychopathology to help explain why some children and adolescents who face adversity early in life go on to do well whereas others do not.[3] While resilience is an important concept in working with transgender youth, most of the literature has concentrated on their risks rather than their strengths, which provides a limited, negative view of the life contexts of transgender youth. However, research on resilience has since shifted its focus to the role of community factors and contextual influences that threaten or support resilience. From this perspective, resilience is comprised of those individual, positive adaptations that individuals make despite experiencing challenging environments.[4] For the purposes of this project, resilience is presented as a muscle that needs to be exercised. After repeated trauma, that muscle can strengthen or become worn out. One's ability to bounce back from adversity depends on the strength of this muscle.

There is significant data published about the health disparities facing homeless transgender people in DC. In 2015, the DC Trans Coalition released *Access Denied: Washington, DC Trans Needs Assessment Report.*[5] With five hundred participants, this is the largest local-level survey of transgender, transsexual, and gender nonconforming people ever conducted in the United States. The report is a statistical portrait of all aspects of life, including income, education, health, housing, experiences of violence, interactions with the legal system, access to identity documents, and the role of LGBT organizations in trans lives.

The data found that transgender people seeking vital services in DC are not safe. Of those who have gone to a shelter, 27 percent were denied access, and of those who had resided in a shelter, 41 percent had been assaulted by residents or staff. LGB serving organizations also provide little safe haven, with 50 percent of those who had sought services experiencing poor treatment during their visit. The mental health statistics were equally grim: 60 percent had considered suicide at some point in their lives, 34 percent had attempted it, and 10 percent had done so in the past twelve months due to the persistent structural violence faced by trans people in DC.[6]

Taking into account the formidable health disparities faced by LGBT people (especially transgender people) in DC, the need to foster resilience was great. While all children experience psychological and social pressures to conform to sexual and gender norms, LGBT youth experience these pressures in their core sense of self. Growing up LGBT in a society that enforces rigid notions of sexuality and gender has implications for safety, sense of belonging, access to adult support, health and well-being, and life opportunities.[7] However, LGBT youth who have developed resilience are better equipped to overcome these challenges.[8]

Casa Ruby is a nonprofit multicultural LGBT center in the Columbia Heights/Petworth neighborhood of Washington, DC, that provides shelter, food, clothing, legal services, and professional development for low-income LGBT people. Casa Ruby was founded by transgender activist Ruby Jade Corado. A native of El Salvador, she fled civil war when she was sixteen years old and has lived in the District of Columbia for the last twenty-seven years. She has devoted the last twenty years of her life to advocacy in mainstream society for LGBT people.

Casa Ruby staff shared with me that the youth needed more constructive, enriching activities to focus on outside of life's difficulties. Sprouting from this expressed need of youth engagement and residential experience, I proposed the idea of facilitating a youth-written and run blog with the residents of Casa Ruby's youth house. I was connected with a twenty-two-year-old resident named Chris, one of the most politically active youth at the house. I spent the next several weeks getting to know Chris, getting introduced to residents, accompanying them during activities and mealtimes, and getting more acquainted with this passionate young man who later became the blog's managing editor.

A native of Lincoln, Nebraska, Chris has had a deep passion for history and politics from a young age. At fourteen years old, he lobbied the then governor of Nebraska David Heineman on issues ranging from LGBT rights to environmental problems. At seventeen, he drafted a petition to remove Article 1 Section 29 of the Nebraska constitution—the state's voter backed Defense of Marriage Act. He traveled the state gathering thousands of signatures for the better part of a year. However, as an out gay teen, he faced significant discrimination in his family and hometown and escaped to DC when he was eighteen. He found Casa Ruby on the internet after living on the streets for several months. When we met, he had been living at the youth house for about eighteen months, making him the longest remaining resident of the house.

In addition to submitting his own entries, Chris recruited youth in the house to submit entries and edited them before sending them to me to post. Jen and Skyler served as "artistic directors," reviewing art entries that were to be posted on the blog. The one Spanish-speaking participant wrote entries in Spanish, and I provided a translation below the entry. All forms of expression were encouraged.

I mean it when I say "youth run." While I served as an advocate on the youth's behalf and as an interlocutor between the youth and the staff, I left it up to the youth to decide how best to tailor this project to their needs.

The project initially served a population of twelve homeless LGBT youth at Casa Ruby's Youth House. However, after six residents moved out of the house and lost contact, that population was cut in half. Participants were between the ages of eighteen and twenty-four.

Given my small sample size and the lack of participation in the post-survey, this did not turn out to be a data-driven project. However, there was a wealth of qualitative information.

One youth responded that they felt as though they had "temporarily taken ownership" of the project. Two youth commented that the blog allowed them to express themselves creatively and voice their opinions. And four of the youth commented in their evaluations that working on the blog allowed them to temporarily focus on something other than the turbulent politics of the house.

Through an opportunity for LGBT homeless youth to blog about their lives, they provided themselves with moments of creativity away from life's difficulties. With enough exposure and support, these gifted queer youth could have a major impact on their communities, while also building resiliency for their own lives and the lives of other queer youth. By reading about other youth that are having similar experiences and knowing that they can also become empowered through self-expression, advocacy, and organizing within their communities, they will be able to strengthen their own resilience.

Arin Jayes (he/they) is a mental health advocate, embroidery artist, craftivist, and urban gardener from Washington, DC. Arin is a graduate of the LGBT Health Policy and Practice Program at George Washington University, the first practice focused, interdisciplinary graduate certificate program in the nation that trains health care leaders and policy advocates on issues relating to the health and well-being of the LGBT community. Arin is currently studying toward his Master's Degree in Clinical Mental Health Counseling at Johns Hopkins University, with the long-term goal of becoming a licensed clinical counselor serving LGBT youth and adults.

Notes

1 K.A. Stieglitz, "Development, Risk, and Resilience of Transgender Youth," *Journal of the Association of Nurses in AIDS Care* 21, no. 3 (May–June 2010): 1–15, accessed June 1, 2019, https://www.ncbi.nlm.nih.gov/pubmed/20347346.

2 Seth T. Pardo and Karen Schantz, "Growing Up Transgender: Safety and Resilience," ACT for Youth Center of Excellence, September 2008, accessed June 1, 2019, http://www.actforyouth.net/resources/rf/rf_trans-resilience_0908.cfm.

3 Stieglitz, "Development, Risk, and Resilience of Transgender Youth."

4 Anneliese A. Singh, "Transgender Youth of Color and Resilience: Negotiating Oppression and Finding Support," *Sex Roles* 68, no. 11 (June 2013): 690–702, accessed June 1, 2019, https://www.deepdyve.com/lp/springer-journals/transgender-youth-of-color-and-resilience-negotiating-oppression-and-bNvZnvu0LU.

5 E.A. Edelman, R. Corado, E.C. Lumby, R.H. Gills, J. Elwell, J.A. Terry, and J. Emperador Dyer, *Access Denied: Washington, DC Trans Needs Assessment Report* (Washington, DC: DC Trans Coalition, 2015).

6 Ibid.

7 Pardo and Schantz, "Growing Up Transgender."

8 Arnold H. Grossman, Anthony R. D'Augelli, and John A. Frank, "Aspects of Psychological Resilience among Transgender Youth," *Journal of LGBT Youth* 8, no. 2 (November 2010): 103–15, accessed June 1, 2019, https://www.tandfonline.com/doi/full/10.1080/19361653.2011.541347.

6

Beyond Duct Tape: Binding for Transmasculine Youth

Preston Heldibridle

Before I had my binder, I was anxious and uncomfortable wherever I went. I felt as if my skin was visibly crawling over my bones and sinew, and everyone who looked at me could see it. After I started binding, I felt normal, like any other average person on the street; being glanced at was no longer a humiliating experience. I'd had no idea I carried that much dysphoria until I had a way of relieving it.

I've been binding for a smidge over two years now, and, overall, my experience with binding is pretty typical for a poor nonbinary kid at a school teetering on the edge of rural and suburban environments.

My first experience with a binder was with one I purchased for my boyfriend to replace one that was hurting him. Though it was too small for me, I couldn't help but try it on before gifting it to him. A lesson was certainly learned that day: I nearly strangled myself with it by accident. This is a common experience for transmasculine youth like me: we have to learn to bind safely.

I wear a commercial binder, which is a specialized article of clothing designed to reshape the chest area and minimize the appearance of breasts. Binding is a method of flattening breast tissue, and is used by many transgender and nonbinary individuals to alleviate dysphoria, anxiety, and depression, improve mood and self-esteem, and help us feel comfortable in our skin. This all helps us function better in work, school, and everyday life. Binding also makes it easier to be perceived as a male in public, and for nonbinary folks not to be mistaken for cis girls. Not all transmasculine people need or want to bind, and some people can't bind for health reasons, but for many of us, the effects of binding are life-altering and drastically improve our day-to-day experiences and, in some cases, save our lives. Unfortunately, there are plenty of hurdles—monetary, medical, parental—that prevent youth from safely performing this affirming practice.

Something that is important for health care professionals to know is that denying access to proper binders is very dangerous in regards to a child's safety. The debilitating effects of dysphoria don't go away because "daddy said no." Tell a parched boy he's not allowed to drink the water in the fridge, and he'll sneak it from the tap. Likewise, if using a proper binder is not an available option, kids will likely, and understandably, turn to alternative and less safe binding methods, which are very dangerous for their health and can set them back for future gender-affirming medical procedures.

Alternative binding methods include taping breasts down with duct tape, wrapping the chest in compression bandages, or using a waist trainer (or other shapewear garments) on the chest. A safe alternative is a medium or high impact sports bra, but the same rules of safe binding apply.

I had to wait months to get a binder of my own, and, in the meantime, I relied on two sports bras and numerous layers of shirts and tank tops. I was able to use this attire to combat my dysphoria to a degree, but even that proved dangerous: it inhibited my breathing so much that I once came close to passing out in a park.

When I was finally able to buy a binder, it was wonderful. As I wore it, I noticed an almost jarring absence of anxiety I had not previously realized I was carrying. Wearing my binder did not make my chest flat, but it did make it much less noticeable, as it is supposed to. I felt so much better as I went about my days and was able to be more present and focused in school and at home, without the constant stress of dysphoria.

When most people think of chest binding, the image of the skinny white kid wrapping their chest in ace bandages or duct tape usually pops into mind. Unfortunately, this scene has been perpetuated throughout media, and kids experiencing dysphoria may be tempted to replicate it with their bodies. Thankfully, in this age of information, most trans youth are relying on information from their peers, friends who bind, or blogs and social media accounts run by trans people. But other transmasculine youth don't know where to turn. Can they ask their doctor? Will their family be supportive? Why wasn't this information covered in health class? These are just some of the unanswered questions that may exist.

For some in our community, the words of medical professionals may not mean much unless backed up by a fellow trans person. They've lost trust that health care professionals know what's best for them due to negative past experiences. This is especially prevalent in rural environments, where trans competent medical care is, unfortunately, harder to find, and misinformation on binding and other trans issues is ever-present.

It's held true enough that the most reliable resources for a trans person are fellow trans people. When I personally researched binding, most of the information I received at first came from the internet (Tumblr blogs, specifically) and trans friends at school. My friends and I certainly helped and supported each other as best we could—more than the adults in our lives were able to—and we learned from the pitfalls along the way.

However, this system isn't perfect. Most trans and nonbinary "mentors" or influencers are young adults ourselves. Additionally, most trans people online are trying to give good examples to the younger or newer folks by making posts with sentiments like, "Make sure to only bind for eight hours at a time!" Unfortunately, it's well known that a lot of us don't follow our own advice and do things like wear our binders all day, because we're already entrenched in our awful habits. Also, we're not doctors, we're youth—but as with so many other LGBT health issues, we are becoming our own advocates to fill a vacuum in our society.

Resources such as LGBT centers are vital for trans youth in cities and often have programs that assist people in getting binders, but those aren't very accessible for those in more rural areas. Transportation is a big issue—community centers are generally near larger population centers, far from those of us in rural environments who don't have access to public transportation, and many youth without vehicles are unable to negotiate rides from guardians or from friends without adult permission.

As previously mentioned, the most dependable source of support for trans kids is often other trans people. In rural areas, trans youth tend to be much more isolated from each other than in more urban and suburban communities. Internet access is an incredibly important factor—especially for those who are isolated from their peers and physical resources, online community is essential for both support and information.

For over a year, that first binder was my only binder. I wore it all day every day, only taking it off to shower. This behavior was quite dangerous; I could have inflicted permanent damage on my body. Over time, my binder wore out and became less and less effective, until there was barely any point in donning it. A trans friend who worked with GC2B (a company that makes binders) learned of my predicament and sent me a new binder for free. Now that binder is the only one I currently own. I try to take it off more regularly than before, but often I forget and leave it on for days at a time, even though I know I shouldn't.

So how does one bind safely? It is absolutely possible for binding to be an overwhelmingly positive experience if done in a healthy manner. Everyone always says "listen to your body," and largely that is good advice. If the binder is uncomfortable or causing pain, something is probably wrong. But as transmasculine youth, we can't always trust that our body will let us know when it is being harmed—many of us deal with pain related to our bodies every day.

Negative effects of binding range from mild to severe, including skin irritation, numbness, trouble breathing, feeling dizzy or faint, chest and back pain, fluid buildup in lungs, exasperated anxiety symptoms, soft tissue damage, weakened muscles supporting the ribcage, hairline fractures, even punctured lungs. Most of these are a result from long-term unsafe binding practices—using alternative binding materials like tape or bandages or binding too tight or too continuously. And severe enough tissue damage can make a person ineligible for top surgery in the future. This is why it's so important that pediatric care professionals can provide medically and culturally appropriate health information to transmasculine patients so we can be informed about safe binding methods. It's also why accessibility, affordability, and insurance coverage for binders is important.

Health care professionals should remind their patients that a binder is not meant to make the chest perfectly flat but to reshape the chest and minimize the appearance of breasts. Most people, including myself, will not be flat when binding. That is okay. Captain America's tits aren't flat either and trans-masculine youth should not take dangerous risks for a flatter chest.

Safe binding practices begin when buying a binder. But cost is often an issue. Safe, commercial binders made by a reputable company should be readily available, covered by medical insurance (before top surgery), and provided to uninsured patients at reduced or no cost.

Binding is a life-changing and even lifesaving practice for so many transmasculine and nonbinary people and can drastically improve quality of life, as long as it's done safely with the right materials. This is why it's crucial to lift as many of the barriers blocking access to binders as possible—so our youth have that chance to thrive.

Preston Heldibridle (he/him/his) is the State Policy Associate with the Pennsylvania Youth Congress (PYC), which advocates for responsible LGBT policy in state government. A 2017 graduate of Dallastown Area High School in southern York County, Pennsylvania, his advocacy as a nonbinary youth largely focuses on trans youth policy. Preston played a critical role in defeating a state bill that would have removed coverage for trans youth enrolled in the Children's Health Insurance Program (CHIP), a major victory for trans youth in Pennsylvania. Currently, Preston is based in Harrisburg and continues doing essential policy work for PYC.

Surviving Suicide

Tyler Titus

I was a freshman in high school. I remember coming upstairs to tell my mother I wasn't feeling well and pleading to be allowed to stay in bed. A short and rushed "whatever you want" was the answer as she continued in a fury to get the rest of my siblings and herself ready to leave on time. I went back down to my room in the basement, passing under the metal beam from which I would fall from my next attempt not even a year after this one. I closed the door to my bedroom, not that it mattered, as no one was home, and even if they were, no one came down to the basement. I laid down in my bed after flipping on my stereo and waited until I knew everyone was gone. Once I knew the house was empty I stood and went over to the wall. My walls, which were once covered with my band crushes, were now mostly bare. There were a few random pictures and posters. I took down a photo that I had won in a balloon-popping dart game at the Crawford County Fair in Meadville, Pennsylvania, and stared for a moment. I clinched my teeth and threw the picture down with force, basking in the sound of shattering glass on the cement floor.

I knelt on my knees and picked up a shard of the broken glass that lay atop the picture. I sat in front of the mirror that my stepmother had given me before she, my father, and half sister moved several states away. Looking back, I don't think it was a gift out of the kindness of her heart, but rather a "What the fuck am I going to do with this?" as she packed their house and bequeathed the problem to me.

I looked into the eyes of my reflection and felt a surge of rage. Through a tight jaw, I whispered, "I hate you." The words embodied my absolute truth. I hated everything held inside that mirror. The tears were sliding down my cheeks and falling into my lap. I pressed the fragment of glass against my wrist. "Fuck you, you pathetic piece of shit," I screamed as I stared at the ceiling.

Every second that I allowed to pass without slicing my wrist sent a pulsating reminder of how pitiful I had become through my veins. The silence and passing time became too much for my senses to process. I climbed to my feet and took off running out of my room and up the stairs. I pushed through the door and fell into the living room.

Tears still rushing, I stumbled into my mother and stepfather's room. I didn't bother turning on the lights. What I was in search of wasn't in the main part of their room. I felt in the darkness for the closet door handle. After a quick turn of the knob the door flew open. My stepfather seldom, if ever, actually hung his clothes so the door was like a pressure release valve and would spew its contents upon opening. I was growing increasingly agitated with my inability to stop sobbing. "What the fuck is wrong with you?" I slapped myself across my face. I dug out a clearing, so I could pull open the gun cabinet. It was never locked. I pulled out the .22 rifle and grabbed a handful of bullets. I fell backwards out of the closet. I felt around on the floor for the loose rounds and shoved them in my pocket. As I was leaving my parents' room I glanced to the wall and saw the picture from their wedding that I had enlarged as a gift for my mother. A surge of guilt ran over my body, and I felt weak. "No, you don't get to take this from me. You don't get to stop me now. Not now, Mom, it's too late. You should have tried before."

I fumbled with the bullets before successfully sliding one into the chamber. I racked the bullet into place. I kneeled and leaned my weight unto the barrel. I clicked off the safety and placed my finger on the trigger. I will never forget the feeling of my heart beating in my chest. The pounding was all I could hear. The rest of the world was silent. My eyes were closed and felt the sensation of metal under my finger. That tiny piece of metal is all that stood between me and my escape. One small movement is all I needed to be free.

My mother's face flashed on the back of my closed eyes. I imagined her finding my lifeless body and shattered face encircled by the pool of dark red blood. I opened my eyes. Furious that my brain was trying to convince me to reconsider. I let out a scream and put more pressure on to the trigger. I pressed harder, knowing that any moment the bullet would find its freedom and I would be granted mine.

The final click never came. The darkness never swept in and the thunderous boom never filled my ears. However, this also meant the internal hell never stopped burning. I don't know what happened. I don't remember the rest of this experience. All I can surmise is that I robotically put all the items I had brought to my room back in their original places and shoved my stepfather's clothes back in front of the cabinet.

The next flash of memory I have of this day was when I crawled into my mother's bed. I remember I was eventually awoken by the sound of barking dogs graciously announcing the return of my family. Later that week, I went back to the gun cabinet and picked up the bullet. I realized what I had done. I had loaded the gun, the same gun I had used dozens of times before, incorrectly. The bullet didn't belong to that gun. Sitting here now, the symbolism is surreal. The bullet didn't fit in the gun just as I didn't fit in my casing. It was the wrong body. All along it was the wrong body.

The bullying in middle school and high school still makes its way into my mind from time to time. I will stare off as I replay the torment over and over. The most haunting memory is the day the three girls chased me from the lunch room into the bathroom. I climbed on top of the toilet, so they could not see my feet. They knew I was in there and stood by the sink. I cried quietly as they laughed and mocked my body, my attire, my voice, and how disgusting it felt to look at me. They would follow me around that school until I graduated and would wait to find me alone. Sometimes, I would stand up to them, but typically I cowered and hid. I would try to tell, to reach out for help, but it never seemed to make it stop so I stopped too.

The kids in school put me through hell. Their words still ring in my ears when the darkness creeps in. However, my peers were not my first bullies. Their words are not the loudest and their wounds did not cut me the deepest.

The darkness that grew within me was a seed planted by the people who were supposed to be fostering self-love. Instead, I learned from a young age that I was defective and had parts of me that should never be shared.

I have been through various forms of treatment, because I didn't want to be different. I subjected myself to criticism, perspectives, and beliefs from religious and traditional communities. I didn't want a life of judgment. I didn't want to fight just to be treated with decency. I didn't want to be isolated. I didn't want to be less than. All I have ever wanted was internal peace. Isn't that all we ever really want? To exist in a space in which we can confidently say we are proud of who we are and at peace with the journey we have traveled.

I survived suicide, and the many factors that lead so many to that point, but this is not the case for all LGBT youth. Today an estimated 60 percent of gender nonconforming and transgender youth, and 40 percent of lesbian, gay, and bisexual youth are actively contemplating or have attempted suicide.[1] They are almost three times more likely to be diagnosed with depression or anxiety due to compromised safety, discrimination, retaliation, rejection, isolation, and abandonment.[2] Shame, rejection, discrimination, and conversation therapy lead a developing brain to inherit a self-perception riddled with disgust, disdain, and hopelessness.[3] These tactics will end the lives of youth who barely had the chance to gain their footing.

There is now an expansive amount of research to show the impact adverse childhood experiences have on a developing brain.[4] We now know that when primary attachment figures inconsistently connect or protect a child will not develop adequate self-soothing skills. This results in increased levels of cortisol in the brain as the limbic system becomes overactivated and over utilized.[5] The child will perceive the world as unsafe and will start to interpret life through these lenses. When a child perceives and receives their surroundings as untrustworthy they will strengthen their ability to protect themselves from it. The end result varies from anxiety and depression to anti-social behaviors and aggression.[6] For me, the experiences took shape in self-deprecation, depression, and emotional dysregulation that sabotaged several of my relationships with friends, family, and partners later in life.

My life experiences created a path for me. A daunting, terrifying, yet beautiful path full of possibility. Once I accepted that I was not broken, I set out to educate and create community for those who knew exactly what darkness felt like, as they lived in it every day. I wanted to send a message to those people who were force-fed fallacies about themselves. I wanted them to know they are not intrinsically flawed. I wanted to create change and compassion. I wanted to be a part of movement that fostered inclusion and understanding rather than formation and perpetuation of fear and ignorance.

For some youth, their soul is too beautiful to be contained by anatomy; we can't shake their shine. Pediatric care professionals can provide encouragement to their trans patients; they should ask about our gender identities and our overall happiness. And policy makers should ensure that schools are safe places for all youth to learn, and that lifesaving trans care is covered for youth by all types of insurance. There is so much love in this world, and this universe needs every one of us. I've learned that it truly does get better and life—crazy, scary, beautiful life—is worth it.

Tyler Titus, father of two amazing little humans, is a licensed professional counselor, advocate, trauma specialist, and elected school board director in Erie, Pennsylvania. Tyler became the first elected openly transgender official in the Commonwealth of Pennsylvania in November 2017. He was appointed by Pennsylvania Governor Tom Wolf to serve as cochair of the Pennsylvania Commission of LGBTQ Affairs. He authored a chapter in *Why I Run: 35 Progressive Candidates Who Are Changing Politics*. In addition, Tyler regularly presents at local and national conferences on the topics of trauma, suicide, and ways that communities can reach out to underserved populations.

Notes

1 Amir Ahuja, Cecil Webster, Nicole Gibson, Athena Brewer, Steven Toledo, and Stephen Thomas Russell, "Bullying and Suicide: The Mental Health Crisis of LGBTQ Youth and How You Can Help," *Journal of Gay & Lesbian Mental Health* 19, no. 2 (May 2015): 125–44; Stephanie L. Budge, Jill L. Adelson, and Kimberly A.S. Howard, "Anxiety and Depression in Transgender Individuals: The Roles of Transition Status, Loss, Social Support, and Coping," *Journal of Consulting and Clinical Psychology* 81, no. 3 (February 2013): 545.

2 Budge et al., "Anxiety and Depression in Transgender Individuals"; Yasuko Kanamori, Jeffrey H.D. Cornelius-White, Teresa K. Pegors, Todd Daniel, and Joseph Hulgus, "Development and Validation of the Transgender Attitudes and Beliefs Scale," *Archives of Sexual Behavior* 46, no. 5 (July 2017): 1503–15.

3 Budge et al., "Anxiety and Depression in Transgender Individuals."

4 American Academy of Pediatrics, "Addressing Adverse Childhood Experiences and Other Types of Trauma in the Primary Care Setting," 2014, accessed June 2, 2019, https://www.aap.org/en-us/Documents/ttb_addressing_aces.pdf; Bessel A. Van der Kolk, "Developmental Trauma Disorder: Toward a Rational Diagnosis for Children with Complex Trauma Histories," *Psychiatric Annals* 35, no. 5 (May 2005): 401–8, accessed June 2, 2019, https://traumaticstressinstitute.org/wp-content/files_mf/1276541701VanderKolkDvptTraumaDis.pdf.

5 Van der Kolk, "Developmental Trauma Disorder."

6 Brian Mustanski and Richard T. Liu, "A Longitudinal Study of Predictors of Suicide Attempts among Lesbian, Gay, Bisexual, and Transgender Youth," *Archives of Sexual Behavior* 42, no. 3 (April 2013): 437–48.

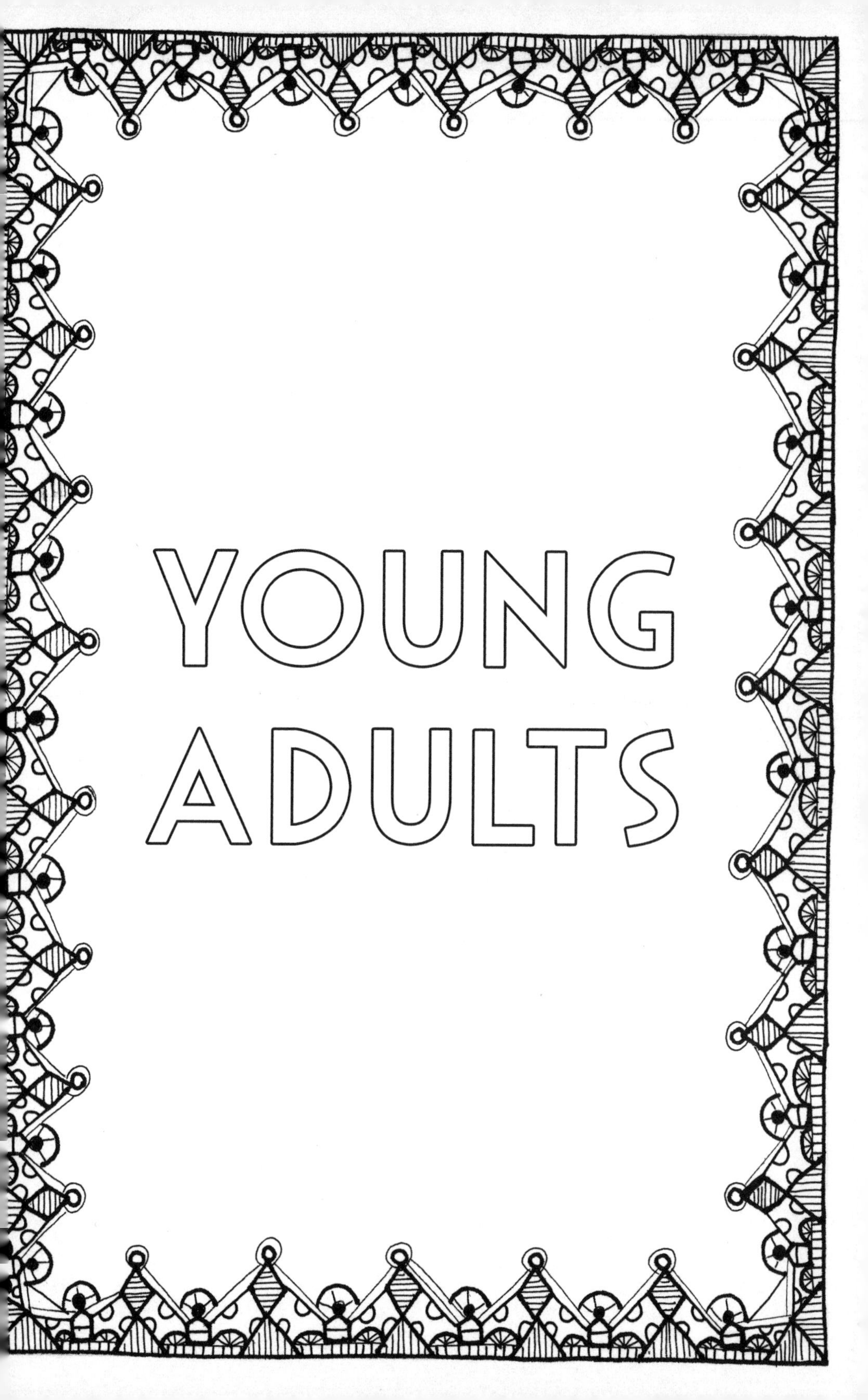

YOUNG ADULTS

8

Sex and Safety in the Digital Age

Jack Harrison-Quintana

When looking for community, companionship, or sex, most young adults head right for their smartphones. Because that's the world we live in today. We cannot talk about sexual health if we don't talk about technology.

When I joined the staff of Grindr in March 2015, the company maintained a prohibition against stating a desire for "unsafe sex" in the text of a user's public profile. The company introduced this rule because of the meticulous care necessary to stay on the right side of the store bureaucracies of Apple's iTunes and Google Play, which maintain strict regulations on both explicit content and apps that might compromise the safety and well-being of their users.

As I write this essay today, however, having spent the last four years as the head of Grindr's team to promote queer health and human rights, I feel less sure than ever what "unsafe sex" actually means.

Part of what has changed is the medical innovation that has expanded users' potential strategies for protecting their sexual health. In addition to condoms, we now have increased access to protective factors like the HPV vaccine for young people and Truvada for pre-exposure prophylaxis (PrEP), the daily pill that prevents HIV.

But the other part of what makes me question this term is the multiplicity of ways queer people's safety can come under attack when they try to connect to their community, whether that be in the form of sex, dating, friendship, or otherwise. My work to make the global queer community safer has forced me to consider so many aspects of safety beyond condoms and even beyond sexual health.

A complete conversation about sexual health should consider the digital dimensions of how sex can be made safer for LGBT people today and, in particular, the role that dating apps and other online platforms are able to play in that endeavor. Drawing on my own experience as a queer man and my professional experience at Grindr, I will move through three areas—sex education, digital and physical safety, and emotional well-being. In conclusion, I will consider the opportunities platforms like Grindr offer to the community and the responsibilities that come with that.

Sex Education

Most LGBT people never receive comprehensive sex education in school or at home, so the lack of information presents many unanswered questions. In November 2017, I launched Grindr's Sexual Health Resource Center (SHRC). Initially, this resource was a collection of twenty answers to frequently asked questions based on the most common questions our team received from app users. It covered questions like: "What is PrEP?" "How can I find my closest STI/HIV testing site?" and "Can I get HIV from oral sex?"

Although the resource originally launched strictly in English, my goal from the outset was to create an expansive multilingual resource that would speak to Grindr's users all over the world in the words our users would best understand.

Today, the SHRC is available in over fifty-six languages. For many of these languages, there is no other sexual health information anywhere on the internet, let alone information that presents sexual health information in a way that centers the LGBT experience.

This was no easy task, even with the necessary funding. It became clear very early on that many professional translators who are heterosexual and cisgender lacked even the most basic vocabulary necessary to speak to our audience. When I first published our Arabic-language resources, I was shocked to hear back from a flood of users in the Middle East that the word that had been used for lesbian was an extremely offensive term that nobody from the queer community would ever dare to say. I realized that this would be a much more arduous process as I struck out to identify and hire grassroots LGBT translators as well as other native speakers from the community who could check their work.

Sexual Health Resource Center Languages

English
Español | Spanish
Português | Portuguese
Français | French
Deutsche | German
Dholuo | Luo
Ελληνικά | Greek
Lugandan
Italiano | Italian
繁體中文 | Traditional Chinese
简体中文 | Simplified Chinese
傳統粵語 | Traditional Cantonese
简体粤语 | Simplified Cantonese
日本語 | Japanese
தமிழ் | Tamil
हिन्दी | Hindi
한국어 | Korean
Bahasa Indonesia | Indonesian
Монгол | Mongolian
ภาษาไทย | Thai
Tiếng Việt | Vietnamese
Pýсский | Russian
Polski | Polish
Кыргызча | Kyrgyz
Тоҷикӣ | Tajik
Lietuvių | Lithuanian
Norsk | Norwegian
മലയാളം | Malayalam
Română | Romanian
Български | Bulgarian
Čeština | Czech
Српски | Serbian
Bahasa Melayu | Malay
Harshen Hausa | Hausa
Ìgbò | Igbo
Gĩkũyũ | Kikuyu
Kikongo | Kongo
Yorùbá | Yoruba
Tagalog
Kiswahili | Swahili
Shona
Setswana | Tswana
አማርኛ | Amharic
Naija | Nigerian Pidgin
Te Reo | Māori
հայերեն | Armenian
isiZulu | Zulu
ಕನ್ನಡ | Kannada
తెలుగు | Telugu
ગુજરાતી | Gujarati
ਪੰਜਾਬੀ | Punjabi
डोगरी | Dogri
বাংলা | Bengali
অসমীয়া | Assamese
Magyar | Hungarian
Somali
Meitei
اُردُو | Urdu
العَرَبِيَّة | Arabic
فارسی | Farsi

The results have been incredible. Of course, many organizations maintain sexual health information. But with 3.8 million unique daily active users from virtually every country on earth, Grindr has proven to be uniquely suited to the distribution of this kind of material.

For example, one of the languages we have featured is Tamil, a tongue spoken by more than seventy million people. Tamil is primarily spoken in one state in southern India, as well as one region of nearby northern Sri Lanka, with a smattering of major migrant communities in Singapore and the Middle East, as well as a quarter of a million people in the United States. Because of Grindr's tremendous global reach and our geolocation-based messaging technology, we are able to send out notifications to the users in all of these areas, ensuring that the resources don't simply sit unread on an auxiliary website, but that we can get it directly to the queer people who need it most. Technology has the power to put sexual health information into the hands of every user of the app.

And the people who use Grindr represent a wide swathe of those who need it most. LGBT and sexual health organizations do the very best they can to get information out to their communities, but we know that there are plenty of queer people who never interact with such an organization and, in fact, may even be scared to go anywhere near them and their resources because of the societal pressures and—in some countries—legal consequences. And yet many of those people still log on to Grindr seeking connection not with activists but simply other community members.

We are also able to integrate these informational resources directly into the user interface of the app itself, giving even more opportunities for users to discover the information. When we added optional profile fields for "HIV Status" and "Last Tested Date," we also included a deep link to these resources next to words that users might not be familiar with like "Positive Undetectable."

Digital and Physical Safety

In November 2017, a popular Lebanese band called Mashrou' Leila performed a concert in Cairo. During the performance, a contingent of activists unfurled a rainbow flag in protest for the liberation of LGBT Egyptians. This set off the most extreme anti-LGBT crackdown Egypt has ever seen, including the arrest of over seventy Grindr users simply for who and how they love.

When I started this job, I underestimated the extent to which my goal of making sex safer for LGBT people around the world would necessitate thinking about situations like this one. But with users logging on from every walk of life, every culture, and every country, I soon realized that many of the safety challenges we as queer people face are about the violence of the world around us. More than seventy countries in the world criminalize gay sex, and just as the app allows people a layer of anonymity when they log on for their own protection, that same anonymity also creates opportunities for our enemies to slip in unnoticed.

The first thing I did with the Product Team at Grindr when we started work on this problem back in 2015 was to identify at the country-level which places in the world would need extra attention because of the risks LGBT people living in them faced. I started with places where the crime of homosexuality carried the death penalty and built up the list from there. For these countries, we decided to turn off exact distances. In other words, the profiles that populate a user's cascade still appear in order of distance but exactly how far away each of them is has been obscured. In major U.S. urban centers, of course, being able to see which users are under a mile from someone's current location is a feature that's core to the app and, in fact, was one of the things that set Grindr apart from its web-based predecessors. But, in a country like Egypt or Iran, we worried that being able to see that someone was within a few meters could give too much information to morality police officers, thieves, gangs, and others who sought to use the homophobia embedded in their legal structures as leverage against individual LGBT people.

What we've found since then, though, is that passive location sharing isn't the key way that people's safety is compromised. In the case of Egypt, again, members of the Cairo police had been pretending to be queer Grindr users and had struck up fake relationships with real gay, bi, and trans people so that in a moment of crackdown they'd already have a relationship with individuals and could easily lure them to meet in person and make the arrest. We've heard these stories of bad actors building trust with queers on Grindr over and over again in different contexts—extortionists in Nigeria, neo-Nazis in Germany, and government representatives spying on the platform in post-Soviet countries. Even staying inside and using the app exclusively for digital pen pal purposes does not always keep users safe. Grindr users have been targeted and forced to pay monthly extortion fees simply based on nude photos or face photos that have identifying LGBT elements.

So in addition to changes we can make inside the app, the conclusion I've come to is that the empowerment of individuals and groups of users is actually the community's own best protection. In the same way that generations of queers have sought to learn self-defense to ward off potential street harassment, queers today can benefit from upgrading their digital security tactics and learning to trust their instincts when they feel that something may be off about a chat or an encounter. That's why we we've employed our network of grassroots LGBT translators to ensure that our basic safety tip checklist can be available in over twenty-five languages, including ones that might otherwise be overlooked for queer resources—languages like Azeri, Hausa, and Bahasa in Indonesia. And although the prospect of encountering a bad actor on the app can be chilling, I am thankful once again to have this network of users so that we do have easy ways to distribute information that queer people may need regardless of their specific app use.

In addition, of course, we've continued to improve the safety options that are built into the app. Through a collaboration with the non-LGBT-specific human rights organization Article 19, which has a focus on digital security, we've been able to conduct research into the specific safety needs of various user groups. We started in Lebanon, and one of the situations we heard most clearly about was that people of Beirut had to pass through government checkpoints throughout the day as they moved around the city. There's not much privacy at these checkpoints, and guards would regularly go through people's phones. Grindr brand recognition had become so widespread that just having the app's mask icon on a home screen was starting to "out" people at these checkpoints, so we built a feature called the Discreet App Icon (DAI) that would allow the user to change the outward appearance of Grindr on their phone, masking it as a notepad app, an alarm clock app, etc. Today, users all over the world, regardless of country, can have access to our Discreet App Icons if they're an Xtra user, and users who live in parts of the world where anti-LGBT violence and discrimination is most pervasive and devastating can access the feature for free.

In a world where homophobia, biphobia, and transphobia still threaten our existence every single day, "unsafe sex" sometimes has nothing to do with barriers for our mucus membranes. Even getting ourselves physically into the space for a date can present challenges that may ultimately impact our health, and consideration needs to be paid to these potential outcomes in order for us to get a true picture of what safety planning looks like for our sex lives.

Emotional Well-Being

Social isolation and loneliness are leading causes of death in the United States.[1] Even beyond the work that I'm able to do through Grindr for Equality, the very nature of the app brings people together in a way that can be lifesaving.

Many of the world's oppressed people share those identities with their family members. For example, in a lot of ways I grew up racially isolated. My mother, sisters, and I were the only Mexican-Americans on the mountain we grew up on in Eastern Tennessee. But despite the general lack of other Latinos around us, I was still born into a family that shared that experience with me, and I always had my mom to look up to as a Latina adult. LGBT people, however, aren't usually born with queer parents. We have to seek out connections to others who are like us outside of our families, putting us at much greater risk of isolation and its consequences.

I don't feel uncomfortable when people call Grindr a sex app. That's actually been my primary use for it in my life. But when we ask our users what they've come for, the answers represent an extremely broad range of connections from friends to dates, roommates, gym buddies, book club members, and digital pen pals. Whether our users find love or sex or friendship, Grindr makes people safer because anywhere in the world, in any country, any city, any rural community—LGBT people don't have to be alone.

Of course, the other side of this is that when we're all together online, we bring with us all the other oppressive baggage we're carrying from racism to ableism and transphobia. And, of course, we're also bringing our own experiences of oppression and turning them on one another in the form of things like femmephobia and body shaming. That's why Grindr launched the Kindr campaign in the autumn of 2018. The concept of the campaign was to give a platform for people who had experienced discrimination and prejudice on the app to share their experiences with the community at large in a video format. It also corresponded with a substantive change in our terms of service that laid out more explicit prohibitions against framing a Grindr profile in terms of what someone *doesn't* want, rather than what they *do* want, especially in terms of social identities and any form of shaming.

Knowing you're not alone in your queer body, knowing there are others out there like you—who share your wants, needs, and desires—is lifesaving. Oppression, racism, and rejection are also emotionally damaging. Technology does not exist outside of our lived experiences, it supplements it. We all must work harder to create social spaces for LGBT people where all are included—that includes LGBT bars, community spaces, and mobile apps. Our communities are filled with our people, and our people can always do better.

Responsibility and Opportunity

Over the past four years of using the app for LGBT health and human rights, there is one question I've been asked over and over again. When people are starting from an assumption that using Grindr is going to increase a queer person's likelihood of contracting an STI, in particular, they often ask me whether we have a responsibility for the sexual health of our users. It's a reasonable question and one that I posed to my first boss the first time I was asked. I wanted to know if he felt that way when he decided to hire me. In other words, was Grindr for Equality born out of a sense of obligation.

He told me he didn't feel that being in the business of connection gave him an obligation. But, rather, what he intended was the incredible opportunities the platform had created for doing this kind of education and movement building for queer people around the world. With 3.8 million unique daily active users on the app from virtually every country on earth, I could see the truth in that, and I also started to feel the excitement of such an opportunity.

Of all the oppressed people on earth, there's no other group as densely digitally networked as LGBT people because of apps like Grindr.

We can all do better to ensure that queer people can experience sexually exciting and healthy lives. We can all do better at providing access to sexual health information. We will be most effective if we use the technology available today to do so. Because that's where the community is. On their smartphones.

Jack Harrison-Quintana, MA, is a queer Latino activist, author, and researcher, currently serving as the vice president for social impact at Grindr and the executive director of Grindr for Equality. His work at the intersection of digital advocacy and LGBT justice has earned him recognition as one of *Foreign Policy* magazine's top geopolitical thinkers of 2016, as well as *Fast Company*'s most creative people in business. Prior to his current position, Jack has worked with the National LGBTQ Task Force, the National Center for Transgender Equality (NCTE), the Global Trans Research and Advocacy Project (GTRAP), and Khemara, as well as on five state and local LGBT-related ballot measure campaigns. Jack has coauthored two books—*Outing Age 2010: Public Policy Issues Affecting Lesbian, Gay, Bisexual, and Transgender Elders* and *Injustice at Every Turn: A Report of the National Transgender Discrimination Survey*. His peer reviewed articles have appeared in the *Harvard Kennedy School Journal of LGBTQ Policy Studies, Transgender Studies Quarterly*, and *HIV Medicine*. A native of Signal Mountain, Tennessee, Jack earned both his BS in International Studies and his MA in Communication, Culture, and Technology from Georgetown University.

Notes

1 American Cancer Society, "Social Isolation Linked to Higher Risk of Death," ScienceDaily, November 16, 2018, accessed June 2, 2019, https://www.sciencedaily.com/releases/2018/11/181116110632.htm.

9

Living Proudly, Living Longer: Advocating for Queer Spaces to be Tobacco Free

Adrian Shanker and Annemarie Shankweiler

They say that the first LGBT community centers were gay bars, and they are right.

Before it was politically or socially feasible for many LGBT people to organize social spaces to build community and to find each other, gay bars in cities small and large had opened their doors.

To be sure, there were numerous problems with pre-Stonewall gay bars—police raids were just one—but they always served as places where LGBT people could find each other. But then, and in many places now, gay bars were literally smoke-filled rooms.

After the massacre at Pulse Nightclub in Orlando, the importance of queer spaces was on many of our minds. We go to gay bars to find community, to feel safe and supported, to be around *our* people. It's the same reason we go to LGBT pride celebrations or LGBT community centers. We want to be in places where we can be free to truly be ourselves. So what does it mean when to be in these spaces we must inhale secondhand smoke for the entire evening?

What's more: tobacco is the leading preventable cause of death in the United States and is a leading cause of twelve common types of cancer.[1] Tobacco is responsible for more LGBT deaths than alcohol, breast cancer, HIV, and gay bashing combined.[2] So what does it mean when our queer spaces, the spaces we go for our safety, are spaces where just standing in the room leads to a less healthy future?

LGBT people start smoking for many reasons, including that we want to feel like we belong.[3] LGBT people are stressed out. Culturally, we experience discrimination, bullying, harassment, and violence at disparate rates[4]—all social indicators for tobacco consumption.[5] Tobacco, like all substances, is a coping mechanism.[6] Research shows that while LGBT people are coming out at younger ages than previous generations, LGBT young adults are achieving lower rates of social well-being than older LGBT generations.[7] The dangers that LGBT people faced in the 1990s are still a relevant and pressing concern, despite the improved legal equality. In a tumultuous political climate where LGBT rights and safety are constantly made to be wedge issues, there is no shortage of a need for a coping mechanism.

For many, an easy to obtain coping mechanism is a tobacco product. The specific tobacco consumption method of choice may have changed over the years but the risks of tobacco consumption have not.

LGBT people have lived through enough shame and stigma related to our health, so as coauthors we are not interested in shaming smokers or making them feel bad about their addiction to nicotine. We frequently hear from community members about how smoking has permeated our culture. Most people are shocked to learn that LGBT people consume tobacco at such disparate rates. Often adults that have been addicted to tobacco products for years tell us how they wish they could go back in time and stop themselves from smoking in the first place. They recount the many times that they have attempted to quit and haven't been able to. We know that advocacy and awareness is the answer, because there are many obstacles preventing LGBT people from successfully and completely quitting.

According to a longitudinal study of more than 1,200 smokers, it can take a person up to thirty quit attempts to quit smoking for a year.[8] We know that it's hard to quit. For a lot of people who are hooked on nicotine, it is especially difficult to quit because everyone they know smokes. Perhaps they've tried to quit three times and haven't been successful. Perhaps they were referred to a tobacco dependence treatment (TDT) provider and had a negative experience because of their LGBT identity. Maybe the actual or perceived cost of accessing nicotine replacement therapy is a barrier to care. Or perhaps the places where they go to feel safe are places where all their other queer friends are smoking.

We want our queer spaces to be places we can all enjoy. And that requires our gay bars, community centers, and pride festivals to adopt tobacco-free policies.

In some communities, it's a given. The laws in some places require all bars or all parks to be smoke-free. Not so everywhere. So in every

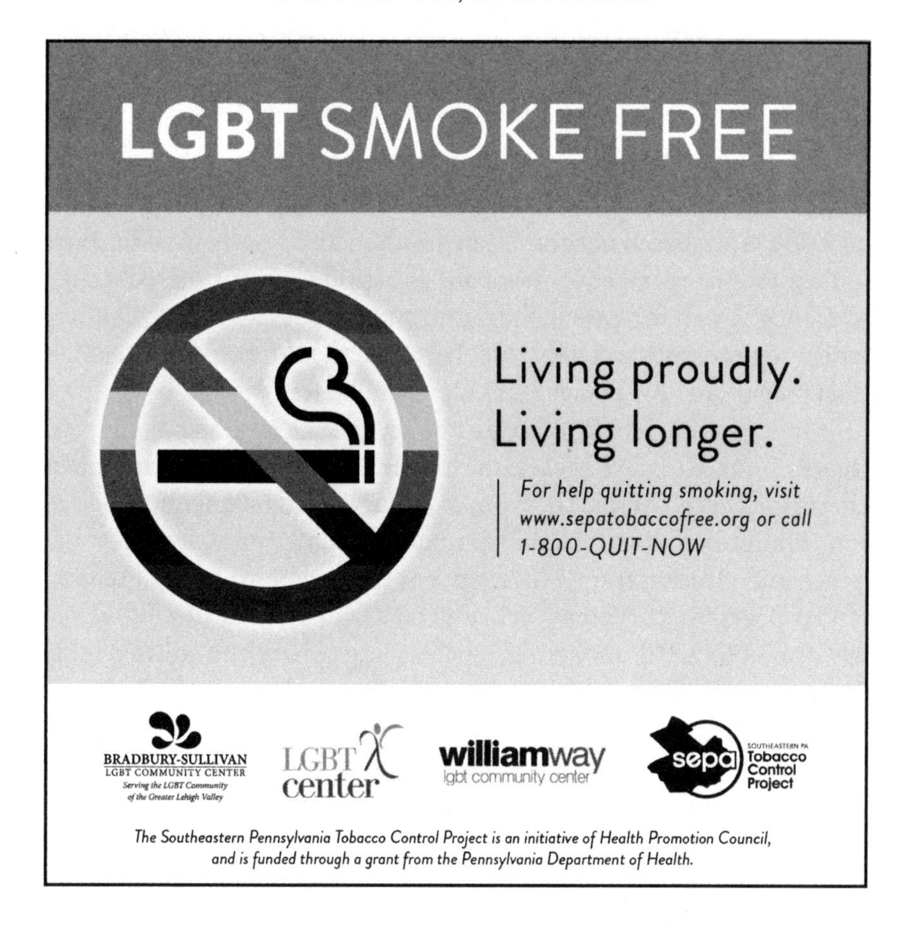

community, those fighting for LGBT health can and should consider working for our queer spaces to be smoke-free—all our queer spaces. The gay bar in the alleyway that's always been a smoke-filled room. The outdoor areas on the campus of the local LGBT community center. The entire route of the pride parade and the annual pride festival. In short: our treasured queer spaces should be places where we can live proudly and live longer.

In Pennsylvania, we've created a successful model that in just four years has led to ten pride celebrations and two gay bars voluntarily going smoke-free. We can achieve this in any community if we want to.

Between 2014 and 2019, Bradbury-Sullivan LGBT Community Center partnered with the Pennsylvania Department of Health, TDT providers, other LGBT community centers, pride celebrations, drag performers, gay bars, and LGBT media outlets to educate our community, create visible clusters of LGBT non-smokers to reduce the social pressure to smoke, and work to enact policy change at numerous LGBT spaces.

We sponsored pride celebrations, and they agreed to a tobacco-free policy for their event: no tobacco sales at pride, no tobacco marketing at pride, no tobacco consumption at pride. The results have been tremendous. An organizer of one of our local pride festivals shared with us that they saw an increase in the number of families with small children attending their pride celebration. Parents had told the pride organizer that they try to only bring their kids to smoke-free events.

It's not enough to simply enact policy change by making our queer spaces smoke-free. We must also educate LGBT community members about the effects of tobacco on our community and on our queer bodies.

Bradbury-Sullivan LGBT Community Center provides direct outreach and education for LGBT student organizations in high schools and colleges, we participate in health fairs with tobacco-free messaging, we provide "LGBT smoke-free" stickers at gay bars and pride celebrations, so non-smokers can identify each other, and we even partner with drag performers to include smoke-free messaging in their acts.

We also provide LGBT cultural competency training for TDT providers, and we partner with these trained providers to have them provide on-site, direct interventions at our local pride festivals for anyone interested in quitting smoking. We can be confident in making referrals to these TDT providers, because we have established relationships, provided training to their staff, and worked with them to ensure that they will offer culturally appropriate health care to their LGBT patients. Since the staff at our state's tobacco-free quitline (1-800-Quit-Now) has also received training on LGBT issues, we also promote the quitline at each pride celebration we partner with. We developed a co-branded campaign, "Living Proudly, Living Longer," in partnership with the Southeastern Pennsylvania Tobacco Control Project, William Way LGBT Community Center, and Central Pennsylvania LGBT Community Center. This campaign has included postcards and billboard placement throughout our region, as well as a long-running ad in each weekly edition of *Philadelphia Gay News*.

The campaign provides social normalization of non-smoking in the LGBT community, encourages a positive reason to quit (live longer) as opposed to a negative outcome for continuing (die sooner), and provides information about the tobacco-free quitline for those interested in quitting smoking.

All the indicators we have seen are that LGBT people want to quit smoking,[9] sometimes we don't know how or where to go. Some well-intentioned health care professionals encourage those trying to quit tobacco to avoid patronizing places where they consume tobacco. But to tell an LGBT person to avoid their local gay bar is socially isolating, especially in small or rural communities. The answer must instead be: let's make the gay bars and all queer spaces smoke-free.

Many LGBT young adults envision LGBT spaces as smoke-free. These are spaces where we can truly be ourselves, where we can find *our* people. These might look like bars, or they might look like LGBT coffeehouses or community centers or pride celebrations. Whether alcohol is present or the menu features an "LGBTea" and rainbow cookie (can't you just see that written on a chalkboard?), the LGBT community will continue to develop social spaces that work for us. A peek into the future would show us that these queer spaces will allow us to thrive. And to do so, they will have to be smoke-free.

Adrian Shanker's bio is on page 207.

Annemarie Shankweiler is an activist for intersectional feminism and queer causes. She earned a Bachelor of Arts in Psychology from Bloomsburg University, where she was a student leader dedicated to empowering women in WISE (Women Inspiring Strength and Empowerment) and creating safe spaces for people of all genders in a local chapter of I AM THAT GIRL. She has worked as a children's counselor, specifically with children affected by domestic violence and sexual assault. She loves music, art, baking, and sipping tea out of a comically large mug with a punchy saying. Annemarie is the Tobacco Education and Outreach Coordinator at Bradbury-Sullivan LGBT Community Center and is currently pursuing a Masters in Art Therapy.

Notes

1 Center for Tobacco Products, "Health Information—Tobacco Use in the LGBT Community: A Public Health Issue," U.S. Food and Drug Administration, July 11, 2018, accessed June 2, 2019, https://www.fda.gov/TobaccoProducts/PublicHealthEducation/HealthInformation/ucm622863.htm; Rebecca L. Siegel, Eric J. Jacobs, Christina C. Newton, Diane Feskanich, Neal D. Freedman, Ross

L. Prentice, and Ahmedin Jemal, "Deaths Due to Cigarette Smoking for 12 Smoking-Related Cancers in the United States," *JAMA Internal Medicine* 175, no. 9 (September 2015): 1574–76, accessed June 2, 2019, https://jamanetwork.com/journals/jamainternalmedicine/fullarticle/2301375.

2 Scout, *MPOWERED: Best and Promising Practices for LGBT Tobacco Prevention and Control* (Boston: Network for LGBT Health Equity, The Fenway Institute, 2012), accessed June 2, 2019, https://www.lgbthealthlink.org/Assets/U/documents/mpowered.pdf.

3 Tamar M.J. Antin, Geoffrey Hunt, and Emile Sanders, "The 'Here and Now' of Youth: The Meanings of Smoking for Sexual and Gender Minority Youth," *Harm Reduction Journal* 15, no. 30 (May 2018), accessed June 2, 2019, https://harmreductionjournal.biomedcentral.com/articles/10.1186/s12954-018-0236-8.

4 Ilan H. Meyer, "Prejudice, Social Stress, and Mental Health in Lesbian, Gay, and Bisexual Populations: Conceptual Issues and Research Evidence," *Psychological Bulletin* 129, no. 5 (September 2003): 674–97, accessed June 1, 2019, https://www.ncbi.nlm.nih.gov/pmc/articles/PMC2072932/.

5 Darla E. Kendzor, Michael S. Businelle, Lorraine R. Reitzel, Debra M. Rios, Taneisha S. Scheuermann, Kim Pulvers, and Jasjit S. Ahluwalia, "Everyday Discrimination Is Associated with Nicotine Dependence among African American, Latino, and White Smokers," *Nicotine & Tobacco Research* 16, no. 6 (June 2014): 633–40, accessed June 2, 2019, https://www.ncbi.nlm.nih.gov/pmc/articles/PMC4015086/.

6 Margaret Rosario, Eric W. Schrimshaw, and Joyce Hunter, "Cigarette Smoking as a Coping Strategy: Negative Implications for Subsequent Psychological Distress among Lesbian, Gay, and Bisexual Youths," *Journal of Pediatric Psychology* 36, no. 7 (August 2011): 731–42, accessed June 2, 2019, https://academic.oup.com/jpepsy/article/36/7/731/986768.

7 Robert M. Kertzner, Ilan H. Meyer, David M. Frost, and Michael J. Stirratt, "Social and Psychological Well-Being in Lesbians, Gay Men, and Bisexuals: The Effects of Race, Gender, Age, and Sexual Identity," *American Journal of Orthopsychiatry* 79, no. 4 (October 2009): 500–10, accessed June 2, 2019, https://www.ncbi.nlm.nih.gov/pubmed/20099941.

8 Michael Chaiton, Lori Diemert, Johanna E. Cohen, Susan J. Bondy, Peter Selby, Anne Philipneri, and Robert Schwartz, "Estimating the Number of Quit Attempts It Takes to Quit Smoking Successfully in a Longitudinal Cohort of Smokers," *BMJ Open* 6, no. 6 (June 2016), accessed June 2, 2019, https://bmjopen.bmj.com/content/6/6/e011045.

9 Research and Evaluation Group at Public Health Management Corporation, *Pennsylvania 2018 LGBT Health Needs Assessment—Summary Report*, accessed June 2, 2019, https://www.livehealthypa.com/docs/default-source/toolkits/lgbt/pennsylvania-2018.pdf?sfvrsn=0&mc_cid=3f3ee7f054&mc_eid=44abda9058.

10

Queer Family Planning: A Remedy to Depression

Kate Luxion

Like most queer people, I don't have a fairytale family; there is a prince for each princess with no substitutions. Fairytales and family units have a socially ordered progression of love, then marriage, then babies. But this progression is stymied by stigma, which shrouds both unmarried and married LGBT youth and young adults, labeling them socially unfit for the role and title of *parent*. Rather than heroic achievers, queer young adults are relegated to cautionary tales without rhyme or reason or consideration of agency or diversity in family constellations.

Depressive Undercurrents: Social Narratives and Families

Growing up in the United States presents a very specific picture of who is considered a valuable member of society. Race, social and financial standing, sexual orientation, and gender identity, among other categories, are intricately woven together into unique identities and experiences.[1] Despite the beauty of innate human diversity, the personification of "model citizen" is most often a white, able-bodied, Christian, middle-class, cisgender man, attracted only to cisgender woman. Companionship then becomes limited to similar race and social standing, with children brought forth through medically unaided reproduction.

Kinship and genetics are often inseparable in legal and medical definitions, reliant on upholding the cisnormative, heteronormative models of family. Queer pregnancy, adoption, surrogacy, and blending families through marriage have been met with bigoted statements disguised as curiosity, questioning queer parents about "the real mother/father." Traditional narratives leave out same-gender and gender-diverse family making and keep us from an accurate telling of humanity's reproductive potential.

Social idealization of who can achieve parental or familial success excludes queer young adults by limiting the accessibility of social benchmarks, such as marriage and children. Lack of representation is compounded by medical policies and practices, embodying social exclusion by erecting barriers preventing queer young adults from accessing health services and reproductive awareness.[2] Social exclusion, stigma, and discrimination all build on top of each other inside the body, increasing depressive symptoms and diagnoses.[3] Social influences of depression are a familiar element of daily life for LGBT young adults, an awareness which mirrors the double-consciousness that W.E.B. Du Bois noted in the early 1900s.[4] A required mental and emotional processing of ever-present images of marriage, families, and happiness that leave LGBT young adults to the wayside when there is no social support to ease depressive symptoms.

Othering of queer young adults is presently done in a manner that supports their need for social support, due to presumed family rejection, without acknowledging their resilience and self-efficacy. In turn, assumed support from LGBT peers negates intercommunity barriers to acceptance of queer parenthood.[5] This places queer young adults at a crossroads with dual sources of shame and alienation from social support. Such an ill-begotten approach also assumes an inseparable connection between health, medical definitions, and the ideal, productive body.[6] What is left are a myriad of reasons why LGBT people shouldn't pursue parenthood without equal attention toward how it can be achieved for those who desire it.

Despite undue, preventable stress from compounding stigma and discrimination, hyperawareness of self and society leads to awareness of unhealthy gender roles and household dynamics found in cisgender, heterosexual homes. To counter the presence of gendered, binary parental roles and responsibilities, queer parenting relationships incorporate planning and undergo clearly communicated expectations.[7] These benefits of partner communication while navigating domestic settings are evident in relationship satisfaction as well, suggesting mental and emotional health outcomes that are equal to or better than their cisgender, heterosexual peers.[8] Regardless of the method of family making, queer family structures support better mental health in the face of greater strain and likelihood of depression.

These academic narratives highlight the resilience of queer young adults. Though queer parenting provides benefits to reduce depressive symptoms and diagnoses, external stressors from unwelcoming and underprepared mental and physical health services need to be addressed.

Needs and Services: Talking Points for Supportive Care

Despite the evidence around LGBT parenting, social narratives and medical and legal barriers still limit access to inclusive sexual and reproductive health services. To make improvements the following recommendations should reduce barriers while opening spaces for LGBT young adults to discuss parenting and reproductive health.

Discussion around family planning for queer young adults must begin before puberty. LGBT children, teens, and young adults are failed brilliantly by current institutional structure of teaching about sexual and reproductive health. The value of queer sex education goes further than knowledge about sexual health, as a lack of knowledge can result in infertility. Sexually transmitted diseases, such as chlamydia trachomatis, can strip the body of fertility regardless of the presence of symptoms.[9] For trans youth who are seeking medical care as part of gender affirmation and general well-being, the discussion of family planning must be presented as a possibility to explore their own agency and provide access to a self-defined future.

The approach currently in place, compliance through silence, results in pervasive and sanctioned sterilization through failure to include LGBT reproduction as a viable and desired option for patients. Thus, holistic sex education and discussion of family planning—including access to contraception and abortion—should be commonplace in physical and mental health care for queer youth and young adults as a means of ameliorating social exclusion.

To facilitate inclusion, gendered medical language should be reconsidered. Binary in its gendering, medical terminology holds up educational privilege that minimizes patient desires and experiences. Proper pronoun usage for patients is becoming more mainstream and should engender the critical analysis of how human anatomy is referenced.

Health literacy barriers and bodily agency both support familiarizing language used by a patient to describe their own body, so they properly communicate their health concerns to a care provider who understands their needs. For example, a preference of "front hole" in place of "vagina" expands vocabulary in a way that retains accuracy without imposing functional expectations of certain bodily openings.

Centering fertility in diverse bodies presents a more realistic picture of reproduction, regardless of sex assigned at birth, sexual orientation, and gender identity.[10] Transgender children and youth should be able to access mainstream representations that allow them to retain reproductive agency while seeking affirming care.

Parenting options should shape the gender affirmation treatment for patients from an early age. This includes clarifying the need for access to gametes—two forms typically gendered under the terms "sperm" and "ovum"—for the purposes of conception. If a trans youth desires to conceive a biological child in the future, gamete collection and storage is one possibility; though it might not be cost-effective or desired for everyone. The following approaches to reproduction and conception should help support queer young adults through the journey of creating a fertility and reproduction plan. Their options should be clearly laid out and considered.

If parenthood embodying the role of gestational parent is desired, there are multiple methods that can be successful regardless of a partner's gamete type—with supportive space for single parents encouraged and enabled as well. Fertilized gametes can be combined either in the body (intrauterine insemination or IUI) or in a clinical setting (in vitro fertilization or IVF). The method of fertilization is one stage, while the medical classification of conception is separate. When one person provides half the gametes and carries the pregnancy it is a single partner conception (SPC). Conceptions that involve both partners can include one providing gametes while the other carries the pregnancy (reception of oocysts from partner, or ROPA), including a subsequent pregnancy of the second partner following an SPC, known as either shared conception (SP) or double partner conception (DPC).

Fertilization and conception are complicated by insurance restrictions, as many policies only validate cisnormative, heteronormative infertility. Sometimes referred to as "biological infertility," this term refers to delays in conception for cisgender, heterosexual couples where two types of gametes fail to become a viable pregnancy. When there is only one gamete type available to a couple outside of cisgender, heterosexual partnerships, this is classified as "social infertility" despite similar fertility constraints occurring in cisgender, heterosexual reproduction. Insurance will cover biologically infertile couples with fewer attempts at conception. For socially infertile couples, the process of accessing insurance coverage of infertility treatments requires more cycles of failed conception of a viable pregnancy.[11] Queer parents-to-be must navigate an already biased health system, mounting costs of care, and ultimately requirements to remain in a system of care longer than necessary due to unfair insurance requirements.

In cases where surrogacy is preferred or required, there are state by state restrictions around the availability of surrogates due to laws around compensation for services. The two different types of surrogacy include traditional/partial surrogacy (where the surrogate provides half the gametes) and gestational/full surrogacy (where all gametes are from external sources). There is a history of lesbian and gay co-parents organizing sperm donations and surrogacy agreements between pairs of same-gender couples, deemed altruistic to resolve compensation laws, in order to form families.[12] Examples include gay fathers as known donors of gametes for lesbian couples or lesbian gestational surrogates assisting gay fathers by carrying the pregnancy.

The complexity of family structures is not limited by legal partnerships, with some biological children being born to couple pairs who chose to co-parent, distributing responsibilities between more than two parents. Legal barriers make queer family making more complicated on paper and in legislation than it is in practice. Conception methods vary, but whether using donor gametes, surrogacy, or a combination, LGBT parents should have clearly stated agreements between parties due to legal barriers that have not caught up with the science of family making.

On the non-medical side of queer family making, case workers and mental health practitioners serve an integral role in the process of fostering and adoption for queer families. Some queer young adults may be referred to a clinical mental health practitioner when seeking assisted reproductive technologies as a procedural test of fitness to parent. These referrals are rooted in outdated, offensive practices that deny care to LGBT parents-to-be.

Additionally, not all parents are granted automatic parental rights at birth, despite having marriage equality, so there may be additional human services imposed upon a queer family that a cisgender, heterosexual family would avoid. Second parent adoptions are often necessary. What's more, state laws sometimes permit county judges to refuse a family's request.

Moving Forward

As the understanding of families and kinship expands to include all of us, the limitations of the current conservative systems become clearer. Biology is not the absolute anchor of kinship, and we will not absolve institutions of bigotry when they use this as their crutch. Families are defined in a myriad of ways, picking up momentum as access and acceptance expands. Whether blended, biological, adopted, chosen, or any variation thereof, a family is made in many ways and should be supported and respected legally, medically, and socially. And when we do so, we will ease the depression plaguing LGBT young adults.

Kate Luxion, MFA, MPH, LCCE, is a genderqueer researcher focusing on LGBT reproductive health and parenting. Luxion serves as executive director of the Journal of Reproductive Justice, a nonprofit organization whose aim is providing inclusive resources and education for queer families and the providers who serve them. When not researching or writing, they serve as a college teacher, advocating for the inclusion and support of queer students. Luxion can also be found working on art with their partner and kiddo.

Notes

1 Lisa Bowleg, "'Once You've Blended the Cake, You Can't Take the Parts Back to the Main Ingredients': Black Gay and Bisexual Men's Descriptions and Experiences of Intersectionality," *Sex Roles* 68, nos. 11–12 (June 2013): 754–67.

2 Dean Murphy, "The Desire for Parenthood: Gay Men Choosing to Become Parents through Surrogacy," *Journal of Family Issues* 34, no. 8 (April 2013) :1104–24; Hongijan Cao, W. Roger Mills-Koonce, Claire Wood, and Mark A. Fine, "Identity Transformation during the Transition to Parenthood among Same-Sex Couples: An Ecological, Stress-Strategy-Adaptation Perspective," *Journal of Family Theory and Review* 8, no. 1 (March 2016): 30–59, accessed June 2, 2019, https://www.ncbi.nlm.nih.gov/pmc/articles/PMC4957560/; lore m. dickey, Kelly M. Ducheny, and Randall Ehrbar, "Family Creation Options for Transgender and Gender Nonconforming People," *Psychology of Sexual Orientation and Gender Diversity* 3, no. 2 (June 2016): 173–79, accessed June 2, 2019, https://www.academia.edu/27991187/Family_Creation_Options_for_Transgender_and_Gender_Nonconforming_People.

3 Ilan H. Meyer and David M. Frost, "Minority Stress and the Health of Sexual Minorities," in *Handbook of Psychology and Sexual Orientation*, ed. Charlotte J. Patterson and Anthony R. Augelli (New York: Oxford University Press, 2013), 252–66; Mark L. Hatzenbuehler, Susan Nolen-Hoeksema, and John Dovidio, "How Does Stigma 'Get Under the Skin'?" *Psychological Science* 20, no. 10 (October 2009): 1282–89. W.E.B. Du Bois, *The Souls of Black Folk* (New York: W.W. Norton & Co., 1999 [1903]).

4 Hatzenbuehler et al., "How Does Stigma 'Get Under the Skin'?"; W.E.B. Du Bois, *The Souls of Black Folk.*

5 Murphy, "The Desire for Parenthood: Gay Men Choosing to Become Parents through Surrogacy"; Cao et al., "Identity Transformation during the Transition to Parenthood among Same-Sex Couples."

6 dickey et al., "Family Creation Options for Transgender and Gender Nonconforming People."

7 Lori E. Ross, "Perinatal Mental Health in Lesbian Mothers: A Review of Potential Risk and Protective Factors," *Women & Health* 41, no. 3 (February 2005): 113–28.

8 Cao, "Identity Transformation during the Transition to Parenthood among Same-Sex Couples"; Ross, "Perinatal Mental Health in Lesbian Mothers"; Rachel H. Farr, Stephen L. Forssell, and Charlotte J. Patterson, "Gay, Lesbian, and Heterosexual Adoptive Parents: Couple and Relationship Issues," *Journal of GLBT Family Studies* 6, no. 2 (April 2010): 199–213, accessed June 2, 2019, https://www.ncbi.nlm.nih.gov/pmc/articles/PMC4460604/; C. Borneskog, C. Lampic, G. Sydsjö, M. Bladh, and A. Skoog Svanberg, "How Do Lesbian Couples Compare with Heterosexual Invitro Fertilization and Spontaneously Pregnant Couples When It Comes to Parenting Stress?" *Acta Paediatrica* 103, no. 5 (January 2014): 537–45, accessed June 2, 2019, https://onlinelibrary.wiley.com/doi/full/10.1111/apa.12568.

9 Andrew J. Para, Stephen E. Gee, and John A. Davis, "Sexually Transmitted Infections in LGBT Populations," *Lesbian, Gay, Bisexual, and Transgender Healthcare* (2016): 233–62.

10 dickey et al., "Family Creation Options for Transgender and Gender Nonconforming People"; Trevor MacDonald, Joy Noel-Weiss, Diana West, Michelle Walks, Mary Lynne Biener, Allana Kibbe, and Elizabeth Myler, "Transmasculine Individuals' Experiences with Lactation, Chestfeeding, and Gender Identity: A Qualitative Study," *BMC Pregnancy and Childbirth* 16, no. 1 (May 2016), accessed June 2, 2019, https://open.library.ubc.ca/cIRcle/collections/facultyresearchandpublications/52383/items/1.0366845.

11 Olivia J. Carpinello, Mary Casey Jacob, John Nulsen, and Claudio Benadiva, "Utilization of Fertility Treatment and Reproductive Choices by Lesbian Couples," *Fertility and Sterility* 106, no. 7 (December 2016): 1709–13, accessed June 2, 2019, https://www.fertstert.org/article/S0015-0282(16)62783-8/fulltext.

12 Katie Batza, "From Sperm Runners to Sperm Banks: Lesbians, Assisted Conception, and Challenging the Fertility Industry, 1971–1983," *Journal of Women's History* 28, no. 2 (Summer 2016): 82–102.

11

Social Service Navigation for the LGBT Community

Anthony Crisci

I live and work in Fairfield County, Connecticut, one of the ten wealthiest counties in the United States. So when I was hired as executive director of Triangle Community Center (TCC) at the age of twenty-five, I did not expect that social service navigation would become our top priority. I was just a few years into my career as a nonprofit administrator, but it didn't take me long to see the need that existed.

TCC is a nonprofit LGBT community center in Norwalk, Connecticut. In its twenty-three years of history, the organization's focus had been offering its facilities to community groups looking for a safe and affirming space to meet. I joined TCC in their transition from an "all-volunteer" organization to one with professional staff. I was young, ambitious, and ready for new challenges, but the stories I heard from some members of our community floored me.

On my second day on the job I received a call I will never forget, in part because I was so unprepared for it.

There was a man on the other end of the line in distress. His voice was cracking and elevated. I could tell he was trying to sound "civil," as so many of us strive to do when interacting with strangers, even when we're in the worst of situations. He asked me if I knew of any LGBT-friendly substance use recovery programs. Before I could scrape together the words to explain to him that I was going to be of little help, he continued with his story. He told me that he was in an abusive relationship, living with his partner on whom he was financially dependent. His partner, he said, was a successful real estate agent despite struggling with addiction. He said that he was the victim of constant emotional and physical abuse, but he knew that if he left his partner he would be homeless and in withdrawal. A dire situation that could easily lead to his death.

I was at a loss. Nothing in my prior LGBT activism could have prepared me for a call like this. None of the volunteers who had been running the organization prior to my hire had told me to expect calls like this one. I searched for local organizations that provided services to survivors of domestic abuse and I looked for local substance use recovery programs. I had no idea which agencies might be LGBT competent and which not. With only two days of work in Fairfield County, I had not yet connected with my peers at other local agencies, and I was unfamiliar with the social service landscape in Fairfield County. To be honest, even though I've retold this story dozens of times, I cannot remember where I referred the person on the other end of the phone to, or even if I made a referral at all. What I do remember is that I ended the call feeling like I had failed. I felt like I had let this person down in their time of need when he called his local LGBT community center for assistance.

The experience left me shaken. But I quickly learned that this call was not unique. In fact, I would soon learn how common calls from local community members in crisis were. TCC set out to change our course to address the social service navigation needs in the LGBT community.

Social service navigation can be described as a five-step process: intake, assessment, referral, follow-up, repeat. Clients first contact the program with what is described as their "presenting need." They are then set up to meet with a social worker, where they complete an intake process that is designed to identify additional needs the client may have. Once the client's needs have been identified, they engage in conversation or "assessment" with their social worker to discuss which of their needs can be addressed at that time. The social worker makes referrals to outside agencies and in-house programs that might satisfy the needs of the client. The client and social worker then agree on a schedule of follow-up meetings, where additional assessments and referrals may be made. Examples of the types of needs that are addressed through social service navigation include housing, food, transportation, domestic violence, and mental health.

In my opinion, LGBT community centers or other LGBT community-based organizations are the optimal location for social service navigation to be offered. Because of negative past experience and numerous barriers to care, LGBT people often feel more comfortable requesting support from a trusted LGBT nonprofit than from a traditional setting.

LGBT community centers are in many ways unique and quirky nonprofit organizations. There are almost three hundred established LGBT community centers in the U.S. alone, and depending on which organization you speak with you might be surprised to learn that each one has a unique perspective on their mission and what programs and services their organization "should" be offering. In large part, this is because community centers are meant to be responsive to the communities they serve. While the LGBT community shares many challenges on a national level, our community's needs vary dramatically on the local level, depending on what state, county, or city the organization is based in and what resources may or may not be available. Most LGBT community centers have developed some kind of service to provide referrals such as online resource directories, training volunteers to make referrals from an established database, or in some cases using paid staff to meet with individuals to assess their needs before making referrals; it was clear to me that very few LGBT organizations were actually funded to do this work, which means they are doing it on top of their other programs and are often unable to dedicate significant staff time to developing a strong social service navigation system.

I couldn't help but feel as though I had stumbled upon a paradox within the LGBT movement. Possibly the most important function that almost all LGBT community-based organizations had in common, was not something that was often discussed, formalized, or funded. While many LGBT centers had funding for program staff to focus on one issue or another, such as a staff person who only focused on domestic violence or a staff person who only focused on mental health, it seemed as though it was very uncommon to have a formalized program that connected these various forms of navigation.

From my experience providing social service navigation, the hardest thing was letting a client know that there weren't services available for them. Whether a client was homeless, had no supportive family, or was dealing with substance use disorder, I knew their experience accessing social services would be much harder as an LGBT person. I knew that they might have a negative or even violent experience at the homeless shelter I was referring them to so they would not have to sleep in the freezing temperatures that night. Or that they might be the only LGBT-identified person in their substance use recovery program, and that they would feel isolated as a result. I also knew that in most cases these were still their "best" options. And while these "best" options are wholly unacceptable, providing navigation to assist community members with their most urgent need is important.

So there is an additional unmet need with social service navigation for the LGBT community. While being LGBT is certainly not a category that automatically qualifies someone for additional services, being LGBT does mean that someone is two to three times more likely to attempt suicide, more likely to experience homelessness, less likely to engage in preventative health care, at higher risk for HIV and STIs, more likely to be overweight or obese, and to experience higher rates of substance addiction, mental health disease, and social isolation. When you look at data regarding some of the more marginalized communities within the LGBT community, such as the transgender community and queer people of color, the list of known health disparities grows even longer. Furthermore, LGBT people rarely experience just one of these health disparities. Many LGBT clients experience comorbidities. The stigma and discrimination that LGBT people experience in their daily lives can certainly amount to a vast array of poor health outcomes. And these outcomes lead to greater need for social service navigation. They are in need of *both* recovery services for substance abuse *and* a safe place to shelter. They are in need of HIV treatment *and* heating assistance. And all of them need to be provided with referrals to agencies that are welcoming.

The fact is that in our current climate, LGBT health disparities are not a new concept. As I began to build relationships with local social service organizations in Fairfield County, I found that many agencies were already trying to make their services LGBT-inclusive and to find methods of effective outreach for engaging LGBT clients who needed their services. While many agencies had the LGBT community on their "target" list, few had any significant engagement with the local LGBT community, and even fewer had an idea of what effective outreach looked like. Perhaps funders hadn't encouraged the mainstream social service agencies to prioritize the LGBT community? Or perhaps these agencies are just overwhelmed by incredible need and limited resources. Either way, the LGBT community was not being prioritized.

At Triangle Community Center, we worked to secure funding to create an action plan for developing our social service navigation program. We knew that creating effective outreach strategies and developing communications channels with our local community was equally important. This new service could only benefit those who needed it if they knew that it existed and how to access it.

In October 2014, we launched a case management program. In the first few months of the program, we did not see clients but instead focused on creating the program itself. We researched policies and procedures and created forms that could be used when working with clients. We talked about intake procedures and started what could develop into a referral database of the known LGBT competent service providers in the area.

By January of 2015, we were ready to begin working with our first clients. In the first year of the program we worked with almost three hundred clients. Our digital outreach strategies were working as were our outreach efforts to other local social service agencies. In fact, many of the clients we worked with in the first year of the program were referrals. Agencies from across the county began reaching out to TCC as a resource and asking us for navigation assistance for their clients. It felt like there was a ton of energy and excitement around the program we had created. Partner agencies did not see our LGBT organization as a competitor, but rather as a collaborator.

With a formalized program, we began receiving invitations to participate in different commissions and advisory boards focused in different areas of local services. These groups included mental health organizations, agencies addressing homelessness, and advocacy organizations. As this program grew, we needed to learn the vocabulary of social service navigation.

The term "navigation" in particular is important. It was one of the services often spoken about at our meetings as being key to addressing some of the disparities our communities were experiencing. It was not enough to simply create information about available resources if the clients who needed these resources were not being navigated to them. I also began to understand the role an LGBT community-based organization can play in a complicated network of social services that had long been established before TCC created its case management program. Instead of being one of the organizations vying to create a new housing complex or a new clinical program, LGBT community centers could just keep doing what was already part of their nature, navigating community members to available resources. Of course, LGBT community centers might naturally take this service to the next level as well by ensuring that they are navigating their clients to the next available LGBT competent resource, which is not always in line with the next available resource someone might be given when working with a non-LGBT agency.

It was an exciting moment when I connected these dots and realized that there was funding available for navigation of services. In 2016, TCC received its first public funding from the City of Norwalk through a Community Development Block Grant for multisector social service navigation and helped ensure that our program could continue to help clients with any presenting needs and did not need to limit itself to just one area. It was soon after that we began a conversation with the Connecticut Department of Mental Health to start a drop-in center program for young adults that also used navigation as a means of intervention for working with clients that needed additional services. In 2018, TCC received its first grant from the Connecticut Department of Housing to provide 211 intakes services and housing navigation.

What had started as an idea and a phone call just a few years earlier had snowballed into a blossoming, successful, and recognized program in Fairfield County. More importantly, hundreds of our local community members were receiving assistance when they called our center. The support we were able to offer to members of our community had completely transformed. One of TCC's first social service navigation clients was a young gay man who was a refugee from Jamaica seeking asylum. He used the center's social service navigation program for about three-and-a-half years while he worked through challenges such as homelessness, seeking asylum, mental health treatment, supporting himself financially, and continuing his education. It was a great honor to see that same client continue his education at an Ivy League academic institution. All of the work that went into creating the social service navigation program for Fairfield County's LGBT community could be summarized in saying that when this client called the center for help, we did not fail.

Anthony Crisci began at Triangle Community Center in September 2013 as the organization's first executive director. During his tenure, Crisci oversaw the revival of Fairfield County's Pride festival, the creation of TCC's social service navigation program, and the inauguration of TCC's LGBT competency training program. Anthony recently transitioned from his position at Triangle Community Center to director of marketing and communications at Circle Care Center in Norwalk, Connecticut. He happily resides in Bridgeport, Connecticut, with his fiancé Will and their household of pets.

12

That Ass Tho! Anal Health for the LGBT Community

Adrian Shanker

I've always been out to all my health care professionals. But I've never had a doctor ask me about my anal health. So I asked my doctor during a physical, "Doctor, you know I'm gay, I'm just curious why you've never asked me about my behavioral risk factors for anal cancer so you would know if I should consider an anal Pap test?" He looked up at me, surprised by the question, and responded, "I guess I didn't think of it—we don't have clear guidelines on this."

That's the problem. My doctor didn't do anything wrong. It's that nobody thinks about it. One hundred percent of humans have an anus. All of us use this essential body part. Some of us find pleasure with it. Few of us ever consider the health of our anus. Fewer of us have ever had a health care professional ask us about it.

Prevalence of anal cancer is thirty-four times higher among men who have sex with men (MSM) populations compared to the majority population.[1] However, anal cancer is rarely discussed between queer male patients and their primary care clinicians. The HPV and Anal Cancer Foundation identifies several risk factors for anal cancer, including HPV, which is widely understood to be sexually transmitted through skin-to-skin contact, including during anal sex with or without condom usage. Receptive partners, without regard to their sex assigned at birth, are at increased risk for anal cancer. HIV positive individuals and anyone with weakened immune systems, such as those with autoimmune diseases or transplant recipients, also live with increased risk.[2] Tobacco is also a leading cause of anal cancer and current smokers have a higher risk factor than former smokers. The LGBT community consumes tobacco at rates much higher than the majority population.[3]

Given the clear behavioral risk factors for anal cancer, one might assume that at-risk populations, such as queer men, would receive regular screenings for early detection and that clinicians would assist patients at risk for anal cancer with knowledge of their anal health. That assumption would be wholly inaccurate.

Dr. Beth Careyva, a primary care physician, shared with me her thoughts for why many clinicians do not ask about anal Pap tests: "For cervical Paps, we have very clear guidelines. Clinicians are unsure what the guidelines are for anal Paps. Many primary care clinicians have never provided an anal Pap test and may be unsure how to order it. Clinicians tend to feel more comfortable when there are clear guidelines and standards of care. In general, there's a significant knowledge gap here in determining who should be screened and at what interval."[4] Her indication of a "significant knowledge gap" is important. In a GLMA white paper,[5] leading LGBT health equity advocate Shane Snowdon wrote, "LGBT inclusion in curriculum plays a critical role in improving health and achieving equity for LGBT patients."[6] A knowledge gap about anal health exists among clinicians at least in part because of the lack of education clinicians received in medical school about LGBT health broadly and anal health in particular.

Primary care clinicians, even many who are well-intentioned and committed to the health of their LGBT clients, may not be asking the most important questions to ascertain the information needed to determine risk for anal cancer and the appropriateness of an anal Pap test. Medical and allied health school curricula should address this knowledge gap by adding content about anal health to their curricula. The Centers for Disease Control and Prevention (CDC) and state departments of health can help too by developing clinical guidelines for anal Pap tests.

The knowledge gap among clinicians is a problem, but the knowledge gap among LGBT health care consumers is equally challenging. The LGBT community has a tradition of being our own advocates. Yet many LGBT health care consumers have never heard of an anal Pap test. According to research by Alison C. Reed et al., "Only 23% of gay and bisexual men had heard of anal Pap tests . . . even fewer (14%) reported having received one. Five men indicated that they had tried to get an anal Pap test but were unsuccessful because their doctor or health care provider did not usually give the test, . . . told them they did not need

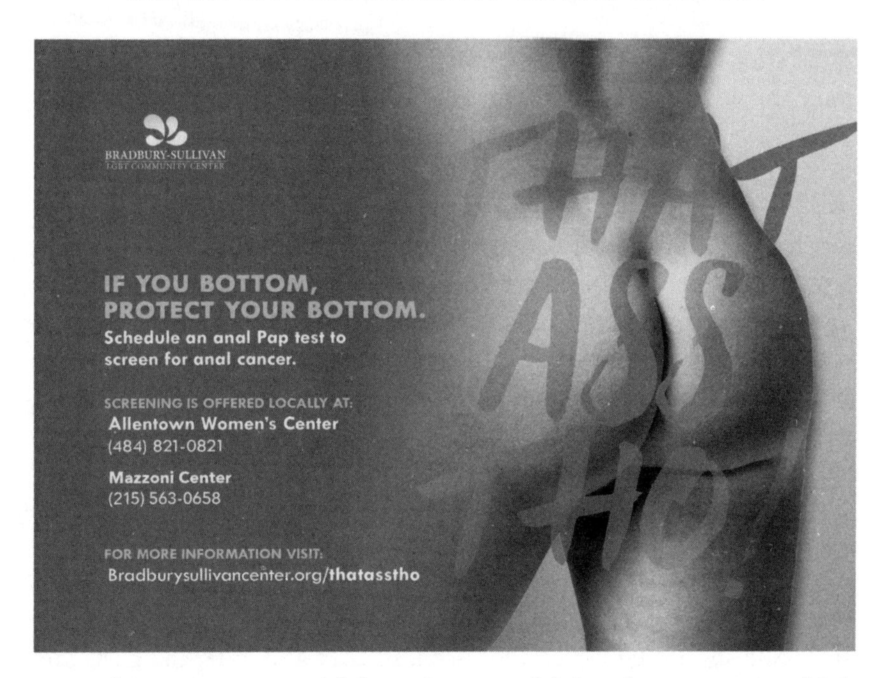

an anal Pap test, or . . . told them the cost of doing the test was too high to justify doing it."[7]

To address the health care consumer knowledge gap, Bradbury-Sullivan LGBT Community Center launched That Ass Tho! an evidence-based health promotion campaign to promote anal Pap tests in the counties served by the center.

That Ass Tho! with the tagline, "If you bottom, protect your bottom" was successful at raising community awareness and has led to two additional clinics in our community preparing to offer anal Pap tests to their patients. But we also heard from clinics that denial of health insurance coverage for their patients to receive the anal Pap test was too great a barrier to overcome.

Reed's research also addressed cost as a significant barrier to care. Reed asked about willingness to receive an anal Pap test at no cost and willingness to pay $150 out of pocket to receive a screening. "Most respondents were willing to accept free screening (83%), but fewer would pay for the test (31%). Willingness to pay for screening was higher among men who reported greater worry about getting anal cancer, higher perceived likelihood of anal cancer, and higher income."[8]

Administering an anal Pap test is easy. Easier than a cervical Pap test—one clinician even said that he finds it easier to administer than a rapid strep test. Yet it's not offered by many clinicians nor is it covered by many health insurers. Under the Affordable Care Act, cervical Pap tests are covered as an Essential Health Benefit (EHB), meaning that there's no cost for the preventative screening. Anal Pap tests are not covered as an EHB, and many insurers don't cover it at all. Health insurers can already predict the cost for anal Pap tests, because they know how much it costs for them to administer a cervical Pap test. Some health insurers are voluntarily covering it, and the rest should follow. And government insurance regulators should mandate parity in insurance coverage between screenings for HPV-related cancers.

Another issue related to the anal health of queer men is oral-anal sex. The health implications stemming from the lack of LGBT-inclusive sex education, medical information from our health care professionals, and the lack of health care consumer knowledge about a common sexual practice among queer men leads us to be unsure what protective factors may exist. What's more, there's a public health reason why this issue should be better addressed. In 2017 and 2018, the CDC and numerous state departments of health identified upticks and, in some cases, outbreaks of the Hepatitis A virus. The increase has largely been centered among homeless individuals and among MSM populations.[9]

Hepatitis A is a communicable disease commonly spread through oral-fecal contact (including oral-anal sex, casually referred to as rimming). Fortunately, there is a safe and effective vaccine to prevent Hep A.[10] However the Hep A vaccine was not routinely provided to children prior to 1999, but many adults think they were vaccinated for it since they were vaccinated for Hep B. Hep A can be spread through sexual activity or contact with fingers or objects that have come in contact with the virus.

There are numerous barriers in place. Many LGBT people report having had a negative past experience from a health care professional, and some fear going to a health care professional as a result. Many LGBT people don't have someone they consider to be their personal doctor; in Pennsylvania, it's almost one in five![11] What's more, many health care professionals lack cultural humility and medical competency regarding the sexual health needs of gay, bisexual, and queer men, and trans women. And as with anal Pap tests, there is a knowledge gap within the LGBT community regarding how Hep A is spread and regarding protective factors, such as the Hep A vaccine.

BRADBURY-SULLIVAN
LGBT COMMUNITY CENTER
If you like
the taste of
peaches,
consider if the Hep A Vaccine is right for you.
#TasteOfPeaches
Sign up for a FREE Hep A vaccination at
Bradbury-Sullivan LGBT Community Center
www.bradburysullivancenter.org/tasteofpeaches

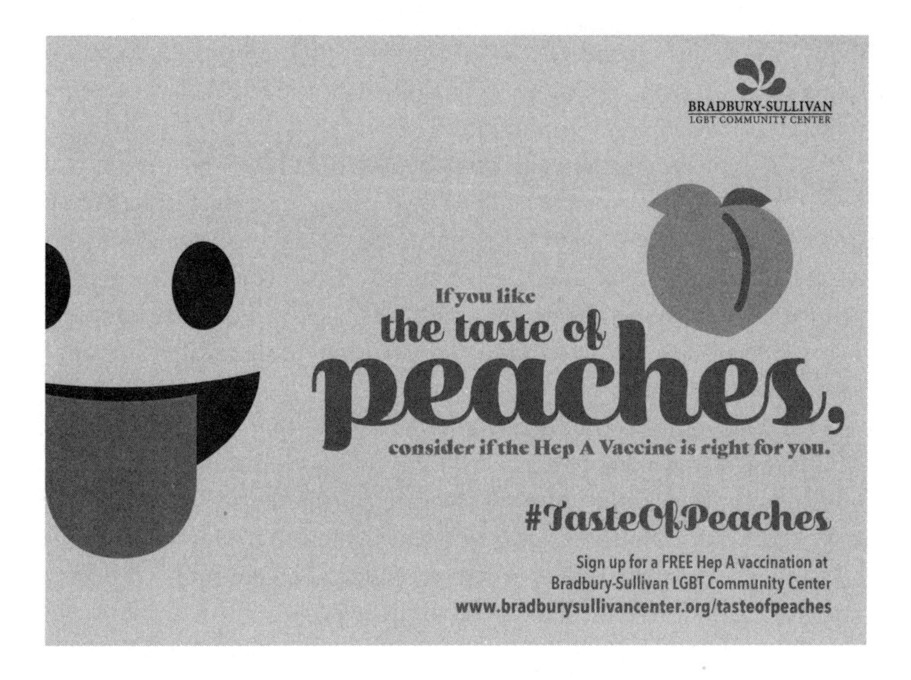

Despite the availability of a safe and effective vaccine that can prevent Hep A infection, many gay and bisexual men have not been adequately vaccinated for it.[12] While rates of Hep A have been on the rise, data available from CDC indicates that only approximately 30 percent of gay and bisexual men are vaccinated.[13]

In response, Bradbury-Sullivan LGBT Community Center launched a health promotion campaign in January 2019 to promote the Hepatitis A vaccine to the LGBT community. The campaign, The Taste of Peaches, is a sex-positive, data-driven campaign to try to reach gay and bisexual men aged twenty-five to forty, to encourage them to get vaccinated. The campaign is co-branded by Grindr for Equality and includes social media, postcards, and in-app messaging to Grindr users.

To further reduce barriers to care, vaccinations are offered in a trusted LGBT space, at Bradbury-Sullivan LGBT Community Center, rather than at a health care facility or community clinic.

But what's unique about this campaign isn't that it is addressing Hepatitis A—there have been many efforts to do so—what is different with The Taste of Peaches is that it addresses Hepatitis A through a culturally appropriate, sex-positive lens. The campaign does not discourage behavioral risk, because doing so would limit sexual satisfaction for many community members. Instead it asks each community member to make a risk-aware decision: "*If* you like the taste of peaches, *consider* if the Hep A vaccine is right for you."

LGBT consumers of health care are tired of judgmental approaches to our health by heterosexist health care professionals and public health experts. Instead, we want to see approaches that incorporate all of who we are, including our sexuality. Risk-aware decision making can do this. But for risk awareness to work, awareness is essential. Unfortunately, many health care professionals are uncomfortable addressing anal health with patients.

Of course, one's anal health involves more than these two issues. Additional issues include access to internal condoms, increased availability and affordability of pre-exposure prophylaxis (PrEP), and sex education curricula that incorporate information about anal health. Like other parts of our bodies, queer people's understanding of our anus and its health needs could be greatly improved.

Queer health activist Michael Scarce wrote "sexual health underpins gay men's individual and collective ability to thrive."[14] If we shine some light where the sun don't shine, our butts and our whole bodies and selves can thrive.

Adrian Shanker's bio is on page 207.

Notes

1 "Behind Closed Drawers," National LGBT Cancer Network, accessed June 3, 2019, 2016, https://cancer-network.org/programs/behind-closed-drawers/.

2 "Living with Anal Cancer/Causes & Risk Factors," *Anal Cancer Foundation*, accessed June 3, 2019, http://www.analcancerfoundation.org/living-with-anal-cancer/anal-cancer-risk-factors-cause.

3 "Tobacco Use in LGBT Communities," Truth Initiative, February 13, 2018, accessed June 3, 2019, https://truthinitiative.org/news/tobacco-social-justice-issue-smoking-and-lgbt-communities.

4 Dr. Beth A. Careyva, telephone interview, July 19, 2016.

5 GLMA (Gay & Lesbian Medical Association), now known as the Health Professionals Advancing LGBTQ Equality, is the world's largest and oldest association of LGBT health care professionals.

6 Shane Snowdon, "Recommendations for Enhancing the Climate for LGBT Students and Employees in Health Professional Schools: A GLMA White Paper" (Washington, DC: GLMA, 2013), accessed June 3, 2019, http://www.glma.org/_data/n_0001/resources/live/Recommendations%20for%20Enhancing%20LGBT%20Climate%20in%20Health%20Professional%20Schools.pdf.

7 Alison C. Reed, Paul L. Reiter, Jennifer S. Smith, Joel M. Palefsky, and Noel T. Brewer, "Gay and Bisexual Men's Willingness to Receive Anal Papanicolaou Testing," *American Journal of Public Health* 100, no. 6 (June 2010): 1123–29, accessed June 3, 2019, https://www.ncbi.nlm.nih.gov/pmc/articles/PMC2866587/.

8 Ibid.

9 "Hepatitis A Outbreaks in the United States," Centers for Disease Control and Prevention, updated December 26, 2018, accessed June 3, 2019, https://www.cdc.gov/hepatitis/outbreaks/hepatitisaoutbreaks.htm.

10 "Gay and Bisexual Men's Health: Viral Hepatitis," Centers for Disease Control and Prevention, updated February 29, 2016, accessed June 3, 2019, https://www.cdc.gov/hepatitis/hav/afaq.htm.

11 Research and Evaluation Group at Public Health Management Corporation, *Pennsylvania 2018 LGBT Health Needs Assessment—Summary Report*, accessed June 2, 2019, https://www.livehealthypa.com/docs/default-source/toolkits/lgbt/pennsylvania-2018.pdf?sfvrsn=0&mc_cid=3f3ee7f054&mc_eid=44abda9058.

12 "Hepatitis A ACIP Vaccine Recommendations," Centers for Disease Control and Prevention, updated November 21, 2014, accessed June 3, 2019, https://www.cdc.gov/vaccines/hcp/acip-recs/vacc-specific/hepa.html.

13 Ronald Valdiserri, "Viral Hepatitis: A Health Concern for Gay and Bisexual Men Deserving Attention," HIV.gov, June 21, 2012, accessed June 3, 2019, https://www.hiv.gov/blog/viral-hepatitis-a-health-concern-for-gay-and-bisexual-men-deserving-attention-during-lgbt-pride-month.

14 Michael Scarce, *Smearing the Queer: Medical Bias in the Healthcare of Gay Men* (Binghamton, NY: Haworth Press, 1999), 171.

13

Addiction and Recovery in the Queer Community

Atticus Ranck

My name is Atticus, and I'm an alcoholic.

I didn't start out that way. I was raised as the third of four kids in a loving, tight-knit, rural Christian family. I didn't grow up around drinking. There were rare occasional family parties where alcohol was present, but my parents never imbibed. I graduated high school without ever going to a party where alcohol was served. I was just that kind of Christian goody two-shoes kind of kid.

Then I realized I was a lesbian, and all hell broke loose.

The church I grew up in was very clear in their stance on premarital sex: *don't do it.* In Youth Group, we were often split into gendered groups, so I was always with the females. At one point during this gendered break out, we were given this analogy: *On our wedding night, we were going to be giving our husbands the "gift" of sex. Our virginity was his present. For every sexual activity we engaged in before sex, a little tear was made in the wrapping of this gift. If we had sex before marriage, the gift would be completely unwrapped. Did we want to give our husbands a gift that was torn or, even worse, not even wrapped, on our wedding night?*

Talk about trauma. The sex education I got in church was heterosexual, heterosexist, and heteronormative. It enforced a rigid cisgender binary system and didn't allow for deviation or any gray areas. The sex education I got in high school was purely anatomical.

So when I started seeing this young woman, I didn't realize I was a lesbian yet or engaging in premarital sex, because this type of thing had literally never been discussed with me.

One night, both my girlfriend and my best friend were staying the night at my parent's house. I kissed my girlfriend, and my best friend caught us. She told my parents, and I was outed. I didn't even get to choose to come out.

My parents immediately split us apart. This started me down a long road of internalized homophobia, questioning my religion and everything I thought I believed in. I also started drinking away the pain.

By the time my senior year started, everybody knew I was a lesbian, but I didn't know I was a lesbian. I was not a popular student, but I was well-liked and had friends in different cliques. I lost all of my friends. I spent the entire year just waiting to graduate. While I never came up with a suicide plan, it was the closest I came to committing suicide. I often thought, "It would be so much easier if I just wasn't here."

I managed to graduate high school by burying myself in my books and my running. Since seventh grade, I had been running cross-country and indoor and outdoor track and field. Running saved me.

I finally graduated and started college. I went to Slippery Rock University, where I was also accepted on their cross-country and track and field teams. The team often drank and partied together. For the first month or two, I didn't drink with them, although I did party with them. A couple of weeks later I finally came out to myself as a lesbian. I wanted to let my newfound friends and teammates know who I really was. I came out to a male teammate, and he helped me come out to the female leaders of my team. In turn, they helped me come out to my teammates. While coming out was awkward at first, everyone was really supportive, and it was a huge weight off my shoulders. I was free to be myself.

At the same time, I started dressing more masculine. I was never a feminine child, but I didn't think of myself as *not female* either. I was a tomboy growing up. When I hit puberty, I tried to be more feminine, but I was also a year-round athlete, so I thought of my look as more "athletic" than "male." There were moments when I tried to look feminine, like wearing dresses, straightening my long curly hair, and attempting to put on eyeliner and mascara, but most often I wore jeans, tee shirts, and my hair in a ponytail.

After I came out at college, I started wearing clothes designed for men. As soon as I put on those male jeans, I never looked back. I suddenly felt more myself and more comfortable. I started to get involved with the LGBT community on campus. Junior year, I was elected president and remained in that position for three years until I graduated.

At first my drinking wasn't problematic. I would drink on the weekends with my teammates after meets, but we partied pretty hard. It didn't take long before I was drinking the nights before races too and showing up hungover. As I started to make friends in the queer community, I would drink with them in addition to drinking with my teammates. I did well enough in my sophomore year of track to qualify for the state meet. That energy and enthusiasm for my sport started to wear off, though.

Then things took a turn for the worse. During the summer between my sophomore and junior years of college, I was raped by a family member.

As a feminist and a gender studies minor, I had learned and discussed sexual assault and rape in the academic setting. I took an academic approach to what happened to me. Finally, though, three months later, I cried about it for the first time. The girl I was dating helped me get into my first mental health counseling sessions. While therapy was incredibly beneficial for me, my drinking was getting progressively worse. The rape was the catalyst that set off my alcoholism.

I started not showing up for cross-country practices. And soon I quit altogether. At the time, I said that my energy was being devoted to my activism, which was true, but the truth was also that running got in the way of my drinking.

It took me five years to graduate college. Most of my friends had left after four years, and I started to feel more isolated during the last year. I started going to the bar more and more frequently. I had a job on campus in the LGBT Center, and one time I showed up still drunk from the night before. I frequently would drink late at night and wake up my roommates. I would often wake up with bruises or other minor injuries, and I usually didn't know how it happened. I was blacking out almost every time I drank.

My therapist encouraged me to see another therapist on campus who had more expertise in addiction, and I agreed. While I was given some skill sets in harm reduction, I didn't see my drinking as problematic yet. I was a successful LGBT leader on campus who was earning high grades and presenting at conferences and speaking at events on and off campus. "I can't be an alcoholic and also be so successful," I thought.

I graduated from college and moved to Florida to start my graduate program in Women, Gender, and Sexuality Studies. I was an out and proud masculine lesbian woman. I had cut my hair short and was wearing exclusively masculine clothing. Early in my time in Florida, I started feeling less and less female, although I didn't know if I identified as male either.

I started slowly dipping my toes into the possibility of transitioning. It really started at the end of my first semester of graduate school when my final paper for Queer Theory was about the prosthetic penis that many trans men use, whether to pee standing up, to pack, to engage in intercourse, or all of the above. I theorized this penis using gender theory and argued that if this prosthetic penis is real to the wearer, it is therefore real. Then I bought myself one and started wearing it. Soon I didn't feel right without it.

I started asking my friends to use he/him/his pronouns only when we were around other friends. Then I found the name Atticus and started asking them to use that name but only in certain situations. By this point, I knew it was becoming much more serious, and I started seeing a therapist on campus about the possibility of transitioning. After reaching our session limit she finally told me that the campus wasn't equipped to handle "cases like mine," and she referred me to a mental health nonprofit agency thirty minutes south of campus.

While I was figuring out my gender identity, my drinking was starting to interfere with my life. I had a graduate teaching fellowship, and I started drinking while I was alone grading student papers. I would frequently show up to my classes to teach either hungover or still drunk. I even missed some classes because of my drinking. When I was out with friends, and they would go home at the end of the night, I would go to my car and pretend to be going home. When the coast was clear, I would go back into the bar and continue drinking. I couldn't walk away from a drink. I didn't drink every day, though, and I frequently went a few days between drinks, because I knew it was becoming a problem and started to feel ashamed. But once that shame wore off, I was back at it.

The typical narrative for many trans people is that they knew they were trans since they were young. That's not always the case, and it certainly wasn't for me. I had a lot of preconceived notions about what it meant to be male. I had sexual trauma related to men. When I first received my penis in the mail after the first semester of graduate school, I was scared of it. It took me a while to realize that this penis wasn't going to hurt me, and it wasn't going to do anything I didn't want it to do. In addition to my sexual trauma, frankly, I found most cisgender men annoying. I didn't like how they took up space in the world by talking over or for women. I didn't like how even the most well-intentioned men hurt the women in their lives. Besides all that, I was proud to be a queer woman! I liked that everybody knew I was a lesbian.

The moment I *knew* I was male came one day in the grocery store. The clerk used she/her/hers pronouns for me, and it finally clicked that it didn't feel right. At this time, I was getting both male and female pronouns, sometimes different pronouns on the same day and in the same outfit; it depended on how the other person saw me. When the clerk used female pronouns on me, it was then that I knew I needed to be seen as the male I had started to feel I was.

In therapy we started breaking down the misconceptions I had about being a man. All my trepidation and hesitation about transitioning was tied directly to my preconceived notions about what it means to be male in our society. I had an "aha" moment in therapy when I realized I could be whatever kind of guy I wanted to be. I could be masculine and male and redefine what that meant. I could treat women kindly. I could be a feminist. I could still be queer and be involved with my LGBT community.

I started medically transitioning to male in December 2013. Unfortunately, the drinking continued, and I actually hit my bottom about five months after starting testosterone. I thought once I started hormone replacement therapy (HRT) that everyone would see me as the guy I am and things would be better. It doesn't work that way. HRT is essentially a second puberty and it takes a few months before anybody can really notice the differences. I was angry early in my transition, because I was doing everything I could to be seen as the guy I am but not everybody was seeing it yet, and I was still too often being misgendered. It was a really low point, and although I was elated to be starting testosterone (T) and was hopeful about my future, alcoholism is a tricky disease, and I was in its grasp.

When I hit my bottom, I was pulled over by the police at 8:00 a.m. I had been out drinking at a bar that closed at 5:00 a.m. I blacked out, so I have no idea when I left the bar or what happened until I came to when the police were at my car. They didn't actually arrest me like they could have, but they did tow my car. That episode was the last straw for my landlord, and he immediately threw me out of the room I was renting in his house. The next day my girlfriend broke up with me. So I was homeless, single, and without a car.

I couch surfed at a friend's house until I found a cheap apartment a few days later. The friend who let me crash at her house told me I should call a mutual friend and fellow grad student, because he didn't drink, and she thought he could be in recovery. I called him and he helped me get into meetings. I got myself a sponsor and started working the steps. By working one day at a time, I haven't had a drink since April 20, 2014.

The person I was when I was active in my alcoholism is vastly different than the person I am now. I like to joke that I used to be an alcoholic lesbian, and now I'm a sober guy. Emerging as male didn't cure my alcoholism, but it certainly helped.

Being sober was hard, though. I didn't know who I was. I didn't know what people did on weekends without alcohol. I didn't know if I could make it an entire weekend without a drink. But I did it. I called my sponsor every day. I started going to the gym. I watched a lot of Netflix. I quit smoking cigarettes three months after I stopped drinking. I continued my therapy sessions. I legally changed my name and my sex. Slowly my beard started coming in. After about eight months on T, I wasn't ever misgendered anymore. I was navigating this scary new world not only as a man but also as a sober person. I didn't often feel like change was happening, but slowly it was.

I completed my graduate internship at the place where I was seeing my therapist. It was an LGBT mental health and social service agency and I was the transgender services intern. Since I had legally changed my name and sex in that county, I was asked to help other trans people legally change their documents. While I had been a student activist and LGBT leader since my undergraduate days, I started to become a leader in the professional world too.

A few months after I graduated, the director of transgender services at this agency moved on, and I was asked to take on the role. I dived into doing the work for my community. I was helping people in ways I had never done before. I let my community guide me.

While I'm an alcoholic, I never attended any addiction treatment programs or halfway houses. Nevertheless, there are times when I'm in the rooms and I feel out of place, even in an LGBT-specific recovery setting. While I was out to my sponsor as a transgender person, I wasn't out to most of the people in the recovery community, and when

I did come out, I was asked a lot of inappropriate questions, even from other members of the LGBT community. I was disappointed in fellow members of my community for not understanding what being transgender meant. I started talking to other transgender people in recovery, and they echoed my sentiments. When I started training addiction treatment organizations, I quickly learned that LGBT people often weren't being properly treated.

At the same time as I started to become passionate about transgender competent care in recovery settings, I picked up a side job as a social media manager for a local therapist and author. He's a gay man who wrote a book, *Lust, Men and Meth: A Gay Man's Guide to Sex and Recovery*, about chemsex in the men who have sex with men (MSM) community.[1] I had never participated in chemsex, but I could relate.

Chemsex is the use of drugs to facilitate sexual activity. The most common drugs used in chemsex are gamma hydroxybutyrate (GHB), gamma butyrolactone (GBL), mephedrone, and crystal meth. The use of these drugs can increase arousal, and they are often used in MSM communities to engage in extended periods of sex.

As I started to learn on my own recovery journey and through my burgeoning recovery activism, I realized how explicitly tied my drinking was to my own identity and feelings of shame. For years, I hadn't engaged in sober first-time sex with anyone. While I could have sex with someone sober, I couldn't the first time we had sex; I always used alcohol to facilitate it. Chemsex is a variation of my own experiences.

I hesitated to be out about being transgender in my own recovery spaces because of the lack of transgender-knowledgeable people. Part of recovery is being able to bring your whole self to the rooms, and I wasn't doing that. I started to feel that not being out entirely about who I was would jeopardize my sobriety. I started talking to other trans people in recovery and to addiction treatment providers and realized how seriously we needed to educate providers so that trans people could recover in safe and affirming spaces.

If a transgender person comes to an addiction treatment center, they need to be placed with the gender with which they identify, even if their legal gender hasn't changed yet. If there is another patient who has a problem with the transgender person in their gendered section, then you move the person with the problem to the single room. This lets the other patients and staff know that we accept and respect the trans person, but that we don't tolerate someone who has a problem with a trans person. Transgender people are just the latest scapegoat. Before, people would have had the same attitude about a gay man sharing a room with them, saying something homophobic or comparing a him to a pedophile or sexual harasser. We don't tolerate those kinds of statements anymore, and we should not tolerate transphobia today. When addiction treatment center staff treat a trans person incorrectly by misgendering them, refusing to use the name that's appropriate for them, placing them with the wrong gender, or placing them in a single room, they are creating a smaller world like the one that helped put that person in the addiction treatment center in the first place—a world of transphobia, violence, disrespect, and micro and macroaggressions. The trans person in the treatment center is there to achieve sobriety and to make their lives better. We can't create the same environment that helped put them there in the first place.

Every person's journey with addiction and recovery is different. This is just one trans person's story, not of my struggles but of my triumph. From sheltered Christian to lesbian and alcoholic to a sober and cigarette-free trans activist. Trans people have so much to offer the world, and it's my hope we can lighten their loads so that they're free to shine.

Atticus Ranck is the Health Program Education Coordinator with the New York State Department of Health AIDS Insitute. He previously worked as the Health Programs and Supportive Services Manager at Bradbury-Sullivan LGBT Community Center in Allentown, Pennsylvania and as director of Transgender Services for SunServe, an LGBT nonprofit mental health center in Fort Lauderdale, Florida. Atticus has trained over one thousand individuals on various aspects LGBT cultural competency over dozens of trainings across the country. Atticus earned his MA in Women, Gender, and Sexuality Studies from Florida Atlantic University and a BA in Creative Writing from Slippery Rock University. In his free time, Atticus enjoys building and restoring furniture and is a huge Harry Potter nerd.

Notes

1 David Fawcett, *Lust Men and Meth: A Gay Man's Guide to Sex and Recovery* (Wilton Manors, FL: Healing Path Press, 2015).

MIDDLE-AGE ADULTS

14

Without Wincing or Clenching: Bisexual People's Experiences with Health Care Professionals

Robyn Ochs

My name is Robyn Ochs. I have identified as bisexual for forty-two years. I'm an educator, an advocate, and a health care consumer.

What do I want my health care providers to know about my experience as a bi-identified person accessing heath care?

The first thing I want them to know is that—even after all these years—the thought of telling a health care professional that I identify as bisexual fills me with anxiety.

I know that the word "bisexual" carries a lot of stereotypes. I'm afraid they will very likely make assumptions about me based on that one word, even if these assumptions are not true. I'm afraid that, as a result, they might not provide me with the best possible health care. I'm afraid they might give me "the look." You know that look. It's the one where your body contracts a bit, you are suddenly no longer making full eye contact with me, and you look like you just swallowed something unpleasant. Are my feelings based on actual bad experiences, or are they based on anticipated bad experiences? *Yes. Both.*

Here are two stories from my own life.

Mind: When I was in my early twenties, I was confused. I was confused about just about everything *except* my sexual orientation. I had already identified as bi for several years, and about that I was 100 percent certain. But I was confused about how to operationalize my bisexuality. There can be an enormous chasm between knowing and being. While it was clear to me who I was, I did not know how to *be* a bisexual person in a binary, heteronormative, and homophobic world. It was clear to me that as a bi-identified person I would not be fully welcome in mainstream society nor would I be fully welcome in lesbian and gay circles.

I was also confused about my career. I was confused about my relationship with my family. I was confused about how to maintain a healthy and successful romantic relationship. I felt tentative and bewildered. Confused. In search of clarity, I decided to see a therapist. I found one on a list provided by my health maintenance organization (HMO).

I saw this therapist weekly for four months. Not once did I mention my bisexual identity. I was afraid. I had no idea what she thought of bisexuality, whether she even considered it a valid, enduring identity. I was afraid she would think I was a lesbian who just hadn't finished coming out. I was afraid she would try to make my therapy *about* my bisexuality. I had heard from other bi friends that their therapists had done such things to them, and I was worried this would happen to me. I could have used some help working through that anticipatory fear and figuring out how to come out and exist in the world as a bi person, but I was too afraid to come out to my therapist. After four months I terminated therapy, having wasted my time and money and her time.

Two years later I decided to try again. This time I selected a therapist who had a connection to Boston's emerging bi community and who I knew identified as bi. By choosing her, I could be certain that my bisexuality would be seen as simply one aspect of my identity. I could be certain that she would not try to help me "finish coming out" as a lesbian. It worked for me. I worked through a number of issues with this therapist. She understood the challenges I faced as a bi-identified person, because they were her challenges too. She got it. The second time's a charm.

Body: In my twenties, during an annual check-up with a new primary care physician, we had the following conversation:

Physician: "Are you sexually active?"

Me: "Yes."

Physician: "What kind of birth control do you use?"

At the time, I was in a monogamous relationship with a woman. I wanted to reply, flippantly, "We use the lesbian method." But I wasn't that brave. I hemmed and hawed and squirmed uncomfortably and finally managed to state that my partner is a woman. It was awkward and uncomfortable.

A couple of years later, that relationship had ended, and I was in a new relationship with a man. I suspected there was a note in my chart saying I was a lesbian, and I finally, awkwardly, told my doctor, "I'm bisexual," and got fitted for a diaphragm.

Is it just me, or are my experiences commonplace? Are my experiences unique? Yes. And no. But, mostly, no.

I bring to my work an intersectional frame. Intersectionality, a term coined by legal scholar Kimberlé Crenshaw, reminds us that each person holds multiple identities, and that people who hold multiple identities that carry social stigma will have specific and distinct experiences of oppression. We experience stigma and oppression in complex, layered, and unique ways. I am white, Jewish, cisgender, able-bodied, educated, a native English speaker, and bisexual. In addition, I have excellent health care insurance coverage, and I live in an urban area that is a major center for medical services, giving me a wide range of health care options. I am fully aware that people with different identities and circumstances may have a profoundly different experience in the health care system. In this way, my experiences are far from universal.

I also recognize the particular challenges of holding an identity not visually apparent. In order to be recognized, I have to actively come out. I can be fairly certain that if I don't, I will be misread. Bi folks share the challenge of holding a nonbinary identity in a culture that leans heavily on binary assumptions.

To gather more information about the specific experiences bi+ individuals have interacting with the health care system, I posted the following invitation on social media:

> If you identify as bi+ and have had a negative (or positive) experience with a health provider related to your sexual orientation, please tell me what happened—today.

I received 132 responses over the course of two weeks. Seventy-eight (59 percent) described negative experiences. Thirty-three (25 percent) shared positive experiences, and 12 (9 percent) provided neutral or mixed responses. Thirteen (10 percent) shared both positive and negative experiences. An additional eight (6 percent) have never discussed their sexuality with a health provider. One respondent wrote: "It doesn't come up." Another wrote: "I would not dream of letting them know!"

Here are a few stories, some of which align with my own experiences and/or fears.

Mind: A nonbinary person, age forty-nine, recounted that they were recovering after a suicide attempt, and a nurse visited them at home. "When I mentioned how biphobia was making my life so hard, she almost jumped back in her seat and made a disgusted face. . . . Months later, and I still have nobody to go to if I have a mental health crisis. Almost every health worker I've seen as an adult is shocked that I'm black *and* bisexual—like it's a thing for white people only. The second most horrible thing was when I saw a gay therapist. He said, 'We'll make a butch lesbian out of you yet!' Like it was a goal for both of us. I felt so insulted and hurt that someone I was vulnerable around would say things like that."

A cisgender bisexual woman, age 25, shared: "I had booked an appointment as I was suffering from panic attacks and anxiety. I was giving the counselor a rundown of my background and mentioned that I was bisexual. He immediately homed in on that despite it being beside the point. He asked me if I was sure, what sexual experiences I'd had, and then tried to blame all my issues on that. I was so uncomfortable that I never went back to him and didn't seek any more mental health help for a number of years. I still don't disclose my sexual orientation to medical providers because of this."

Body: A bisexual/pansexual man, age twenty-seven wrote, "A [primary care clinician] I used to see explained they did not support my lifestyle and told me that they would prefer I get tested for HIV before any appointment and bring the results. They were that panicked and also homophobic."

I heard from a bisexual/asexual female, age twenty-eight, who said, "When she learned I was bisexual, my physician assumed I would be sleeping around a lot and insisted on putting me on hormonal birth control, which wreaked havoc with my depression and anxiety. She did not understand when I insisted that I was asexual and didn't need or want it. She told me 'even hand stuff counts' and wrote the scrip."

There were many different stories shared, and some themes emerged. I'll share excerpts of representative negative stories first, grouped by theme, and then positive ones.

Negative Experiences

Heterosexual Assumption

"[M]idway through a scheduled checkup with my pediatrician (I was seventeen), during the bit where I usually get asked questions about my sleeping habits and household safety and so on, my doctor asked, 'You like boys, right?' I said, 'Yes,' but I wasn't sure how to non-awkwardly add that I also like girls, so I didn't." (cisgender bisexual female, age twenty-five)

Homosexual Assumption

"In more than one instance I had therapists tell me that I'm actually gay, or even after I've corrected them still refer to me as gay." (bisexual male, age fifty-seven)

Making It All About Bisexuality

"The therapist attributed my bisexuality to me having difficulty with commitment/making decisions." (bisexual female, age thirty-three)

"One therapist seemed more enamored with the details and mechanics of my relationship with my partner than in addressing the issues that drove me to therapy in the first place." (bisexual female, age forty)

"I think therapists get really hung up on queerness. My current therapist is great, I do like her a lot, but we focus a lot on my gender identity and romantic/sexual identity. My coming out *is* a part of my struggles with mental illness, I can't deny that, but it's not all of it. I often find that entire sessions are focused on my bisexuality rather than what I'm actually there for." (nonbinary bisexual and queer person, age twenty-one)

Not Believing in Bisexuality

"I once had a therapist tell me that I said I was bisexual simply because I craved attention and needed to feel like a victim." (bisexual woman, age forty-three)

"A psychologist claimed my depression stemmed from my identity as bi because 'that isn't a real thing.' She told me to go to a 'great campus lesbian group' and gave me the number. I ran the group." (agender/woman, age forty-four)

Sex Shaming (Perceived or Real)

"I went for routine STI testing and was asked why I was requesting these tests. I informed [the nurse] that my partner and I were in a non-exclusive relationship and we were both committed to monitoring and maintaining our sexual health. The nurse then responded, 'Why don't you just have one partner and not worry about testing?' A little shocked, I responded, 'I'm bisexual and my lady and I have at times had other male lovers.' The nurse heightened my shock by telling me, 'Well *that's* kinda risky, don't you think?' I asked her how many straight nonmonogamous men had been in for routine STI testing. When she answered, 'Hardly any,' I pointed out that she was probably missing the real risk factors." (bisexual male, age fifty-five)

Conflating Identity and Behavior

"After disclosing my sexual orientation, a physician wrote in my file that I was 'high risk' under the sexual health section of my health chart. In this appointment, we didn't discuss anything that should have indicated this information—I was on birth control, using condoms, and at the time was in a monogamous relationship. The fact that I was labeled high risk because of being bisexual plays into stereotypes and made me feel so ashamed." (bisexual woman, age twenty-five)

"I went for an STI checkup and was told that because I was bisexual that I was at high risk, no matter what my sexual practices were." (bisexual male, age forty-eight)

"I was married to a cis-male, and when I was asked about my sexual history and I mentioned my girlfriend, the nurse practitioner sneered and said it was good I was straight now." (asexual/bisexual/demisexual person, age forty-nine)

Provider Is Uninformed

"After seeing that I had marked 'bisexual' for my sexual orientation on the medical history survey, he commented that it was out of the ordinary. I responded that I didn't find it that odd. He then said 'being attracted to men and women, that's pretty rare.' He then ordered several tests for STDs, despite my (true) assertion that I was not sexually active and had not been for some time." (bisexual male, age thirty-two)

Overt Anti-LGBT Beliefs or Behavior

"A nurse practitioner told me 'if you want any help changing your lifestyle, let me know.'" (queer/pansexual/bisexual person assigned female at birth, age twenty-nine)

Nonresponse

"With both a therapist and a physician I had the same experience—they simply did not know how to respond when I said I was bisexual. I got responses of 'Hmmm. . .' raised eyebrows, meaningful nods—but in neither instance did they actually know what this meant or how to respond. So, we never spoke about it again. I was too exhausted to try and educate either of them. No outright biphobia, but a simple lack of understanding—and no desire to educate themselves." (anonymous)

Hands Over Ears

"As soon as I said I was bisexual, [my health care professional] stopped making eye contact and absentmindedly flipped through the pages of the file in front of him. Then he said, 'Well that's not any of my business,' got super uncomfortable and left without giving me more details. It was absolutely his business as my gynecologist." (bisexual/pansexual woman, age thirty-two)

Anticipating a Negative Response

"I recently switched insurance and have yet to schedule an exam, even though I'm due for a [cervical Pap test]. I'm nervous that my new doc won't be as understanding and accepting [as my last one]." (female bisexual, age thirty-three)

Positive Experiences

Most of the positive stories followed a similar thread: "didn't bat an eye when I told them I was bisexual."

"I had a great experience with a doctor at the health center in college, who asked, 'How many sexual partners have you had?' And when I stumbled over 'It depends how you define sex,' she asked, 'How do you define it?'" (cisgender, bisexual/queer woman, age thirty)

"For the first time in my life, I was asked if I was sexually active and with which genders. When she asked me that, not assuming I was only with men, I cried and thanked her for it because it was the first time that'd ever happened to me." (bisexual woman, age thirty-three)

"I initially gendered all my past partners as male because I wasn't sure what [my therapist] would think about bisexuality. When I corrected and told her the truth, she also took the time to sensitively unpack my internalized biphobia and go through my traumatic memories of bullying and judgment for my sexuality. I have also noticed that she has taken the time to educate herself more about the struggles of bi people—which she previously admitted to not knowing much about." (cisgender bisexual woman, age thirty-four)

"During my first appointment, my doctor asked the question 'do you have sex with men, women, or both?' And I replied 'all', because 'both' would imply two genders, which isn't correct. She silently finished the chart and about 15 minutes later she said very thoughtfully that with my answer, I was making her rethink that question that she had been asking for her entire career. She thought she was being inclusive but understood now why 'both' would be problematic and decided she was going to ask 'men, women, or all?' from now on." (bisexual/queer cisgender woman, age twenty-five)

So my wish is that my current and future health providers will see beyond the binaries and remember that people who are attracted to people of more than one gender exist, are plentiful, and may use a wide variety of labels (or none at all). I want them to know that identity and behavior are not the same thing. I hope they will remember that regardless of how open and informed they are (or believe themselves to be), their patients will likely fear a negative response, and this may well impact their comfort and honesty in the patient-provider relationship. Any proactive steps health care professionals can take to mitigate this fear—using inclusive language (e.g., same-sex relationship instead of lesbian or gay relationship, LGBT family instead of gay family, respecting and using a person's chosen identity words, having LGBT- and bi-affirming materials in their waiting and exam rooms, educating themselves—can increase the likelihood that patients will be comfortable and honest with their health care professionals.

What do bisexual people want? Samati Niyomchoi sums it up beautifully in the March 15, 2016, issue of *The Advocate*: "I'll see my doctor in a few weeks, for a routine visit. I'm glad I'm out to my provider. We'll talk about my sex life openly, freely, and without judgment. I'll get the results of my routine HIV and STI tests from my last appointment, and I'm confident the results, whatever they may be, will be delivered with care and compassion. At the end of the day, that's what any bisexual, any LGBTQ person, and human being deserves: access to an affordable, nonjudgmental medical provider, who will offer and provide tests as requested and needed, without wincing or clenching when we are honest with providers and ourselves."[1]

Robyn Ochs is an educator, speaker, grassroots activist, and editor of *Bi Women Quarterly* and two anthologies: the forty-two-country collection *Getting Bi: Voices of Bisexuals Around the World* and *RECOGNIZE: The Voices of Bisexual Men*. An advocate for the rights of people of *all* orientations and genders to live safely, openly, and with full access and opportunity, Robyn's work focuses on increasing awareness and understanding of complex identities and mobilizing people to be powerful allies to one another within and across identities and social movements. Robyn was recently named by *Teen Vogue* as one of "9 Bisexual Women Who are Making History." She is the recipient of Campus Pride's Voice & Action Award, the Bisexual Resource Center's Community Leadership Award, PFLAG's Brenda Howard Award, the National LGBTQ Task Force's Susan J. Hyde Activism Award for Longevity in the Movement, and the Harvard Gender and Sexuality Caucus's Lifetime Achievement Award.

Notes

1 Samati Niyomchoi, "A Bi Guide to Doctor's Appointments," *Advocate*, March 15, 2016, accessed June 23, 2019, https://www.advocate.com/commentary/2016/3/15/bi-guide-doctors-appointments.

15

Gender, Cancer, and Me

Liz Margolies

I don't have cancer. So far. That is a good thing.

But over a ten-year period, I accompanied four queer women to edge of the cancer cliff, and then watched them all tumble over it and die. These were not just four people I knew and lost; they were four of my favorite people on this planet. Adria, Ruth, Jo, and Shirley all died of ovarian cancer in their fifties. During that same decade, three other friends were treated for breast cancer. What are the odds of this? Slim, I would have thought, but it turns out that this massive loss is not the product of bum luck or a poor choice of friends on my part. This is what health disparities look like in real life. When I was forced to understand this by falling face first into my grief and rage, I set out to tell the world. I was in my fifties too.

Please don't pull out that inaccurate trope that "cancer doesn't discriminate." I've heard it way too many times, and I've lost my patience with explaining. Yes, rogue cells are rogue cells, but we cannot tease out the lives of the errant cells from the social conditions in which the whole body lives. The stress and stigma of living as sexual and gender minorities in this culture absolutely contributes to poorer health and increased cancer risks in LGBT people.[1] For example, my community uses tobacco, alcohol, and other drugs at substantially higher rates than the general population, all coping strategies.[2] As a group, lesbians and bisexual women are said to have the densest cluster of breast cancer risks: increased tobacco and alcohol use; lower likelihood for having a biological child before age thirty; and higher incidence of obesity.[3] Then, instead of being hypervigilant about cancer screening, LGBT people avoid the health care systems, due to substantially lower rates of insurance coverage and previous negative experiences in hospitals and doctors' offices.[4] Our cancer screening rates are dismally low, especially for transgender and gender nonconforming people.

It is highly probable that our community has a higher incidence of cancer, given the increased risk factors and decreased screening rates, but since no national cancer registries collect information about sexual orientation or gender identity, we remain buried in the vast data on file. Luckily, a few states, like California, ask about gender identity in their health surveys, giving us a glimpse of the national picture. And here we see that 14 percent of lesbians and 17.6 percent of bisexual women report having had cancer at some point (vs. 11.9 percent of heterosexual women).[5]

Once diagnosed with cancer, LGBT people are thrust headlong into the health care system, ready or not, and consistently show worse outcomes to treatment, resulting from provider and systemic bias, and lack of provider training in LGBT culture and health. The "worse outcomes" I reference are not measured by differences in scans or blood work or even mortality. It is wholly possible that the multiple providers who have treated LGBT cancer patients might not know about their dissatisfaction with care. In fact, they may not even know who their LGBT patients were, as the hospital forms probably didn't ask about sexual orientation or gender identity, and the providers were unlikely to ask directly. Some LGBT people do come out on their own to their doctors, nurses, PA's, technicians, etc., but those people are twice as likely to be partnered.[6] LGBT patients who are single, who live in a community where the only cancer center is in a Catholic hospital, or who fear that coming out will alienate the doctor who holds the power to save their life keep their silence and often go to medical appointments and chemotherapy alone.[7]

There is some research on LGBT cancer survivors and here is what we know: LGBT cancer survivors have lower satisfaction with care than heterosexual cancer survivors, even controlling for demographic and clinical variables.[8] Breaking it down, lesbians and bisexual women are more than twice as likely to rate their current health as fair or poor, compared to their heterosexual counterparts,[9] gay and bisexual men report more psychological distress after surviving cancer than their heterosexual peers,[10] and gay men with prostate cancer report significantly worse bother scores,[11] worse mental health functioning, and greater fears of the recurrence of cancer.[12]

I was trained as a clinical social worker and spent most of my professional life as a psychotherapist. I considered myself an activist, however, changing the world one soul at a time. This was not facetious; I meant it. I came of age in the radical seventies, steeped in the anti-psychiatry movement that questioned the "science" of psychology, exposing its roots in social control. Focusing on women, my peers and I were challenging the use of medication and psychotherapy to manage the justifiable anger women felt about their restraints on their social/professional/sexual/financial options. Valium was too often the offered cure for women who balked at their roles as homemakers. What passed as "psychology" and was taught in every university class was based on white male experience and, therefore, the ways the rest of us differed in our experiences and feelings was understood as immature at best or pathological at worst. So to make women's experience central to our understanding of "people" was and still is a radical act. We took the field of psychology and centralized the experience of gender, recognizing that it is not biologically determined but dynamic and a reflection of the cultural, economic, and political times we live in. The experience of gender permeates every aspect of our existence—what we eat, what we tell ourselves when we look in the mirror, how we walk, and where we go.

To improve my skills after graduate school, I enrolled in a feminist therapy program, occurring well outside of the traditional psychoanalytic training institutes—those grand, historical, and hierarchical structures that mimic our cultural problems all too well. Older white men held most of the positions of power. The program I chose was small and collaborative. It offered no certificates or recognized credentials.

Later, I became a member of the Feminist Therapy Institute, a ragtag national group of incredibly intelligent women psychotherapists from across the country who supported each other to create both feminist psychology theories and practice, publishing multiple books that remain most proudly on my shelves today. I worked my way up to president at the turn of the last century. FTI no longer exists; that is both a sign of our achievements in opening up the field of psychology and a sad conclusion, as fewer young people identify with this label.

Those early years of feminist therapy may seem quaint today, as identity politics has changed so much. But at the time we were participating in the model of how disenfranchised groups, minorities, and the underserved create alternative spaces and take care of each other. When politics, traditions, and mainstream culture disavow our experience, we find power by huddling with our own. We've seen that with the Civil Rights Movement of the sixties and the early years of the AIDS epidemic, where LGBT people banded together to take care of our sick and fight for access to better treatments. In fact, we see this now in cancer care, as LGBT people disproportionately serve as caregivers to others, not just our partners and friends but also our parents and even our neighbors.[13]

Somewhere in the late 1970s, I also came out as a lesbian. On the surface, this may seem like a matter of choosing women as sexual and romantic partners, but, for me, the greater upheaval was the explosion of my sense of my own gender and a newfound freedom to express it. While feminist theory greatly expanded my sense of possibilities, alongside strong repeated slaps of recognition at social injustices, becoming queer redefined what being female was for me, broadening the category to allow me to embrace, for the first time in my life, my skinny, flat-chested, no-makeup appearance. To be clear, I never doubted that I was female, or, more accurately, that I *wanted* to be female, but my body type, super-delayed puberty, and lack of interest/ability in the "women's arts" of hair and dress had always made me feel like a female imposter. Suddenly, I wasn't an ugly duckling woman; I was a radical lesbian swan. I chopped my hair off and purchased my clothes from the boys' racks. For the very first time, I felt unapologetically and truly female. In addition to my feminist therapy community, I now also had a supportive and celebratory gang of political dykes.

And so I grew older. And so I came to have four lesbian friends die of ovarian cancer. In response, in 2007, I rose from my psychotherapy chair and started the National LGBT Cancer Network. I knew nothing about how to start an organization, having been a psychotherapist for thirty-five years, tucked into a quiet and private room every day. But I knew how to find out what I didn't know. I took my dog to Barnes and Noble and planted us both on the floor in the Nonprofit Books aisle. I read all the "how to start a nonprofit" books. I also talked to as many LGBT people as I could, those with cancer and those on the treatment end. I asked them all what they thought needed to be done. It's one thing to locate a problem; it's another to figure out how to fix it. Across the country, there were several small lesbian breast cancer programs, and I contacted them too, but not one of them addressed all cancers and all subpopulations of the LGBT community. Some were just for lesbians, and others were just for breast cancer. In my novice days, it already seemed clear that all subpopulations of the LGBT community shared many similar health disparities and challenges in survivorship.

I had to bone up on the whole field of cancer, beyond my friends' experiences. I learned that cancer is usually conceptualized as a continuum, from prevention through diagnosis, treatment, survivorship, to end of life. This is often a helpful way to think about the disease, as most professionals focus on only one phase, passing their patients on, sometimes with the help of navigators, to the next group of treatment providers. So, for example, the radiology department may find a breast lump, refer the patient to a surgeon for removal of the lump, who then passes the patient on to oncologists for chemotherapy, with multiple interactions with social workers and nurses and technicians along the way.

I found out, however, that, for LGBT people, the traditional cancer continuum is not adequate for addressing our experiences. In addition to the stress and fears that all people diagnosed with cancer feel at nearly every turn, LGBT people face additional and repeated challenges in all phases of the cancer continuum: decisions about disclosure and fear of discrimination. "Coming out to one's provider" is not a one-time decision. The dance of "Should I tell?/Will I be asked?" is repeated over and over again across the continuum. Cancer patients have dozens of providers, from oncologists to phlebotomists to social workers to MRI technicians. Each disclosure is a real risk for people who feel like their very survival depends on both the good will and skills of their providers.

Just as psychology is not the unbiased science of mind and behavior, oncology is not a medical and unbiased science of the diagnosis and treatment of cancer. Similar to our process when redefining psychology, when I had to study the standard texts, but then hold them up against the data of women's experience, in order to understand how cancer is lived by LGBT people, I had to listen carefully to what real queer people told me. My four dead friends were all white Jewish middle-class lesbians. Their experiences were quite varied, but still that revealed very little about what it means to be gay, trans, a person of color, poor, rural, and/or young and face cancer treatment in this country. All of our identities determine our cancer experience, and there is great diversity among us.

I learned that cancer treatment is profoundly gendered. To claim it is about science and surgery and chemotherapy, all neutral terms, is to miss the gendered environment in which treatment is offered and the impact of treatment on one's felt sense of gender. One's sense of gender also shapes cancer treatment decision-making.

Let's look at breast cancer as an extreme example, where treatment nearly always includes surgery. Losing one's breast(s), partially or fully, by choice or necessity, can change one's embodiment of gender. For transgender cancer patients, the option of a bilateral mastectomy may be perceived as a gender-affirming surgery; the butch lesbian may welcome the option of smaller breasts but may not want to be perceived as transgender by going flat; and the young femme-identified patient may choose reconstruction. In nearly no cases are health care providers tuned into this gendered aspect of medical decision-making. They are, therefore, not able to help the patients choose the best surgery for their lives, not just their health. Still, despite pressure from surgeons to elect one of the multiple types of breast reconstruction, more and more sexual minority women choose to go flat.[14] While some prefer to live without breasts, others are willing to do so, rather than have multiple surgeries to construct new breasts, each carrying some risk and longer recoveries.

The same goes for hair. Many chemotherapies cause hair loss; how women choose to handle baldness is one of cancer's largest challenges, as women are socially defined by having long hair, or at least some hair. It is a primary signifier of femaleness. Here, too, I've found that many sexual minority women forgo the use of wigs, choosing to expose their baldness or wear baseball caps. This impacts their sense of felt gender, as well as the way they are perceived in the world.

If not the health care providers and hospital social workers, who is there to help sexual minority women adapt to the changes in their gender post-treatment? Most cancer surgeons are totally unaware of the significance of patients' felt sense of gender as a guide to treatment decisions. Women and transgender patients are left to their own informal social supports. The "look beautiful, feel beautiful" programs nearly always focus on wigs, makeup, and prostheses, a trio of little significance to the lived experiences of most LGBT breast cancer survivors. A sixty-year-old white lesbian interviewed by my colleague Mary K. Bryson said, "When I'm walking around on the street and I meet other people, I'm not sure I'm being perceived as a woman. People must say to themselves, 'Is this a woman, a man, a boy, or an old man?' When I look at myself in the mirror, I ask myself 'Who am I?', 'Am I still a woman?' And the answer is 'Yes.' I am still a woman for my partner. And for the friends who know me . . . I am a woman. For society, I may be more of a trans person. I understand my road. It's a road that includes removal of my breasts. I don't feel like putting on a prosthesis and then a bra. It's so uncomfortable. I don't want that."[15]

Finally, the "pinking" of breast cancer, the unrelenting forced optimism, expressed with pink ribbons and teddy bears, is the most ubiquitous and largely invisible gendering of the breast cancer experience. It was no surprise to me that many people in our national survey expressed disgust at the cuteness and girlyness of the campaign.[16] When they refused the pink gifts in the hospital, they were perceived as ungrateful or cranky; no one seemed to understand how anathema the objects were to their sense of gender identity and expression, how wrongly they expressed their hopes and fears of breast cancer.

It's been a long career and I am still going. I am sixty-five years old. I don't have cancer. So far. That is a good thing. But I know it may not always be so. Age is the greatest risk factor for cancer, meaning that the older we get, the greater our odds of contracting cancer of some kind: ovarian cancer, breast cancer, or other less gendered cancers. As queer people's lives go, mine has been one with less discrimination than most; I am white, professional, and live in New York City, a safe and welcoming place for people like me. I also have access to healthy foods and outdoor space to exercise. I do what I can to stay slim and strong.

I wonder sometimes what it will be like for me to have cancer. Will all my professional work and research serve to make my cancer experience less stressful? Is forewarned forearmed? Will I be bolder in my demands for the respect and care I want from both my providers and the health care system? What if I am forced to choose, as many are, between using the "best doctor" (who's an asshole) or the young, less experienced queer doctor? What will I do?

Most probably, like everyone else, I will wing it. I'll bumble, I'll cry, I'll be afraid, and I'll forge on, one way or another. I'll lean on my friends for support. I'll be tired. I will be angry. I will experience cancer like I experience the world: as a woman, as queer, and as white. My experience will be gendered. My experience will be mine.

Liz Margolies, LCSW, is the founder and executive director of the National LGBT Cancer Network, the only U.S. program that focuses exclusively on the needs of LGBT people with cancer and those at risk. Margolies is a coauthor of multiple peer reviewed articles, several based on the Network's original research on LGBT cancer survivors. After having developed a nationally recognized cultural competence training curriculum for health and social service providers, Margolies travels the country training large hospital systems and speaking at conferences. As a result of her work for the LGBT community, Margolies was chosen as one of the OUT100 in 2014.

Notes

1 Gilbert Gonzales, Julia Przedworski, and Carrie Henning-Smith, "Comparison of Health and Health Risk Factors between Lesbian, Gay, and Bisexual Adults and Heterosexual Adults in the United States: Results from the National Health Interview Survey," *JAMA Internal Medicine* 176, no. 9 (September 2016): p. 1344–51, accessed June 3, 2019, https://www.ncbi.nlm.nih.gov/pubmed/27367843; James M. Grant, Lisa A. Mottet, and Justin Tanis, *Injustice at Every Turn: A Report of the National Transgender Discrimination Survey* (Washington, DC: National Center for Transgender Equality, 2011), accessed June 1, 2019, https://static1.squarespace.com/static/566c7f0c2399a3bdabb57553/t/566cbf2c57eb8de92a5392e6/1449967404768/ntds_full.pdf; Jillian C. Shipherd, Shira Meguen, W. Christopher Skidmore, and Sarah M. Abramovitz, "Potentially Traumatic Events in a Transgender Sample: Frequency and Associated Symptoms," *Traumatology* 17, no. 2 (June 2011): 56–67.

2 Sean Estaban McCabe, Tonda L. Hughes, Wendy B. Bostwick, Brady T. West, and Carol J. Boyd, "Sexual Orientation, Substance Use Behaviors and Substance Dependence in the United States," *Addiction* 104, no. 8 (August 2009): 1333–45, accessed June 3, 2019, https://www.ncbi.nlm.nih.gov/pmc/articles/PMC2975030/; John Blosnich and Kimberly Horn, "Associations of Discrimination and Violence with Smoking among Emerging Adults: Differences by Gender and Sexual Orientation," *Nicotine & Tobacco Research* 13, no. 12 (December 2011): 1284–95.

3 Antronette K. Yancey, Susan D. Cochran, Heather L. Corliss, and Vickie M. Mays, "Correlates of Overweight and Obesity among Lesbian and Bisexual Women," *Preventive Medicine* 36, no. 6 (June 2003): 676–83, accessed June 3, 2019, https://www.ncbi.nlm.nih.gov/pmc/articles/PMC4174334/; Catherine Meads and David Moore, "Breast Cancer in Lesbians and Bisexual Women: Systematic Review of Incidence, Prevalence and Risk Studies," *BMC Public Health* 13, no. 1127 (December 2013), accessed June 3, 2019, https://bmcpublichealth.biomedcentral.com/articles/10.1186/1471-2458-13-1127.

4 Ninez A. Ponce, Susan D. Cochran, Jennifer C. Pizer, and Vickie M. Mays, "The Effects of Unequal Access to Health Insurance for Same-Sex Couples in California," *Health Affairs* 29, no. 8 (August 2010): 1539–48, accessed June 3, 2019, https://www.healthaffairs.org/doi/full/10.1377/hlthaff.2009.0583; Gilbert Gonzales and Lynn A. Blewett, "National and State-Specific Health Insurance Disparities for Adults in Same-Sex Relationships," *American Journal of Public Health* 104, no. 2 (February 2014): e95-e104, accessed June 3, 2019, https://www.ncbi.nlm.nih.gov/pmc/articles/PMC3935660/.

5 Barbara G. Valanis, Deborah J. Bowen, Tamsen L. Bassford, Evelyn A. Whitlock, Pamela Charney, and Rachel Anne Carter, "Sexual Orientation and Health:

Comparisons in the Women's Health Initiative Sample," *Archives of Family Medicine* 9, no. 9 (September–October 2000): 843–53; Diane L. Kerr, Kele Ding, and Amy J. Thompson, "A Comparison of Lesbian, Bisexual, and Heterosexual Female College Undergraduate Students on Selected Reproductive Health Screenings and Sexual Behaviors," *Women's Health Issues* 23, no. 6 (November 2013): e347–e355.

6 Charles S. Kamen, Marilyn Smith-Stoner, Charles E. Heckler, Marie Flannery, and Liz Margolies, "Social Support, Self-Rated Health, and Lesbian, Gay, Bisexual, and Transgender Identity Disclosure to Cancer Care Providers," *Oncology Nursing Forum* 42, no. 1 (January 2015): 44–51, accessed June 3, 2019, https://www.ncbi.nlm.nih.gov/pmc/articles/PMC4360905/.

7 L. Margolies and N.F.N. Scout, *LGBT Patient-Centered Outcomes: Cancer Survivors Teach Us How to Improve Care for All* (New York: National LGBT Cancer Network, 2013).

8 Jennifer Jabson and Charles S. Kamen, "Sexual Minority Cancer Survivors' Satisfaction with Care," *Journal of Psychosocial Oncology* 34, nos. 1–2 (January–April 2016): 28–38, accessed June 3, 2019, https://www.ncbi.nlm.nih.gov/pmc/articles/PMC4916952/.

9 Ulrike Boehmer, Xiaopeng Miao, and Al Ozonoff, "Cancer Survivorship and Sexual Orientation," *Cancer* 117, no. 16 (August 2011): 3796–3804, accessed June 3, 2019, https://onlinelibrary.wiley.com/doi/full/10.1002/cncr.25950.

10 Jabson and Kamen, "Sexual Minority Cancer Survivors' Satisfaction with Care."

11 Bother scores are based on a self-administered questionnaire that measures how bothersome symptoms are to the person. See, for example, Michael P. O'Leary, "Validity of the 'Bother Score' in the Evaluation and Treatment of Symptomatic Benign Prostatic Hyperplasia," *Reviews in Urology* 7, no. 1 (Winter 2005): 1–10, accessed June 3, 2019, https://www.ncbi.nlm.nih.gov/pmc/articles/PMC1477553/.

12 Charles Kamen, Karen M. Mustian, Ann Dozier, Deborah J. Bowen, and Yue Li, "Disparities in Psychological Distress Impacting Lesbian, Gay, Bisexual and Transgender Cancer Survivors," *Psycho-Oncology* 24, no. 11 (November 2015): 1385–91, accessed June 3, 2019, https://www.ncbi.nlm.nih.gov/pmc/articles/PMC4517981/.

13 National Alliance for Caregiving and AARP Public Policy Institute, *2015 Report: Caregiving in the U.S.* (Bethesda, MD/Washington, DC: National Alliance for Caregiving and AARP Public Policy Institute, 2015), accessed June 3, 2019, https://www.aarp.org/content/dam/aarp/ppi/2015/caregiving-in-the-united-states-2015-report-revised.pdf; Gary J. Gates, "In U.S., More Adults Identifying as LGBT," Gallup, January 11, 2017, accessed June 3, 2019, https://news.gallup.com/poll/201731/lgbt-identification-rises.aspx.

14 Rachel Lynn Wandrey, Whitney D. Qualls, and Katie E. Mosack, "Rejection of Breast Reconstruction among Lesbian Breast Cancer Patients," *LGBT Health* 3, no. 1 (February 2016), 74–78.

15 Mary K. Bryson, Evan T. Taylor, Lorna Boschman, Tae L. Hart, Jacqueline Gahagan, Genevieve Rail, and Janice Ristock, "Awkward Choreographies from Cancer's Margins: Incommensurabilities of Biographical and Biomedical Knowledge in Sexual and/or Gender Minority Cancer Patients' Treatment," *Journal of Medical Humanities* (November 2018): 1–21, accessed June 3, 2019, https://www.academia.edu/38139363/Awkward_choreographies_from_cancers_

margins_Incommensurabilities_of_biographical_and_biomedical_knowledge_in_sexual_and_or_gender_minority_cancer_patients_treatment.

16 Margolies and Scout, *LGBT Patient-Centered Outcomes.*

16

"Laura Is a Transgender. Didn't the Surgeons Do an Amazing Job?"

Laura A. Jacobs

"Laura is a transgender. Didn't the surgeons do an amazing job? You'd never know," said the specialist to the intern, as I sat, fully clothed, on the exam table. I heard the sanitary paper crinkle as my legs dangled over the edge, awkwardly childlike.

Every trans-identified person I've ever met has experienced it:[1] a medical interaction during which we felt fetishized or insulted, when a provider used insensitive or inappropriate language, where a professional pried for information not relevant to the clinical issue. Rather than encouraging a bond, these moments only amplified the resistance.

My sleep had progressed from poor to worse. I spun in the bed, drifting into the beginnings of sleep, but then never falling further or maybe waking abruptly and being unable to fall asleep again. The ragged, inconsistent rest I did get was hardly enough; each day I swam through fog, barely alert. My work suffered, and I had little energy to enjoy life.

I began seeing Dr. B., an ear, nose, and throat doctor and sleep specialist several months earlier to evaluate allergies, medication side effects, environmental issues, diet, stress, or anything else. We determined that the adenoid and turbinate membranes inside my sinuses were swollen and possibly had been for quite some time. My tonsils also were inflamed. As a result, my breathing was uneven, I sniffled and struggled to get enough oxygen, the airflow interrupted by enlarged tissue shrinking the passages. Minor surgery scheduled for a month or two ahead would open the airway. But we were there for a presurgical consultation, and never in any of our visits had I been undressed.

I wanted to list the annoyances as my consciousness spun: no one is "a transgender." We are "transgender people," beings who, for a quirk of biology, spirituality, or a yearning to explore the human experience through the lens of gender, felt the desire or need to live in a way other than how we were born. Some of us have altered our bodies, others not. We each have thought at length about how to define our identities, and our language choices are deeply personal, intended to reflect our nuanced understandings of our selves. We also are not a monolithic group solely defined by our genders but a diverse set of individuals for whom gender is just one of the many facets of who we are. A simple question about what terminology was best would have been appreciated.

She also disclosed without asking permission. I had indicated my transness on the intake forms and had mentioned it in the initial evaluations, unashamed. But other than the possibility that estrogen had affected my sinuses (something we ruled out), my being trans was irrelevant and telling the intern served no purpose. Instead the doctor "outed" me without consent or need. Raising the issue at the beginning of the interaction framed my identity to the intern solely in terms of my gender, as though I was little else.

While language and disclosure issues were irksome, her other comments were even more disaffecting.

The "amazing job done by the surgeons" remark was less about my identity than about my body, but I had never undergone surgery to my face, so she could only be referring to the neck down.[2] I felt an onrush of anxiety: Why were my genitals the subject of an examination of my sinuses? Not only had she just told the intern "what I had down there" but "what I used to have," and that I'd made decisions to be altered from one to the other. Why? What business was it of the intern? The room suddenly felt far too warm.

Did breaking this social convention mean I could have made similar comments about her body? Asked whether she had undergone labiaplasty, surgery to restore the hymen after she became sexually active, or breast augmentation? Sexual organs are private, shared with intimate partners and generally few others, and transgender people retain the same privileges of confidentiality as everyone else. Her unnecessary disclosure came with no consideration of how I might feel.

I also had difficulty understanding the purpose of her compliment. She seemed to be praising me for "passing," for looking conventionally attractive as a woman despite my male past, but this struck me as equally odd and inappropriate, as though passing was a triumph.

I resist labels. When pressed I identify as both trans and genderqueer, defining myself as "dapper" or as "someone transfeminine doing my own version of female masculinity," whatever that may mean. I dress in slacks and buttoned shirts, often ties and vests, and have not worn lipstick or a skirt in a decade. I enjoy playing with gender norms, problematizing them to highlight the implicit stereotypes of our culture. I do not personally feel "born in the wrong body."

Some of us crave passing and do everything we can to minimize the "tells" of our pasts: we remove or grow hair, dress to minimize or accentuate body features, undergo hormone treatments and surgeries to alter our bodies to align with norms of the gender with which we identify. For me, passing had never been the goal and many are unable to pass due to their body type or lack of financial resources to access services. What were her assumptions?

The confrontational activist in me was incensed. How dare she? "You haven't seen anywhere touched by the surgeons. Show me yours and I'll show you mine," I wanted to say. I felt pressured to educate, to make clear her ignorance so as to aid her next trans client and to shame her before the intern.

Instead I said nothing, startled and afraid of being seen as hostile by someone who would soon wield a knife inside my throat.

This was my example, one of many. But ask any trans person, and they will tell a similar tale of a doctor prying about genitals while being treated for a broken arm. Or of a psychotherapist focusing on one's trans identity when you are seeking help with work stress or family dynamics or overall depression. (We can be depressed for reasons utterly unrelated to being trans.) Or of hearing providers snicker after exiting the exam room. We need the care but too often feel demeaned in the process.

Many factors contribute to this perceived lack of safety.

Power disparities are inherent in all medical relationships, and there is a long history of transgender people being objectified by providers.[3] Western medicalization of trans identity coalesced in the 1950s around Dr. Harry Benjamin, and transness was understood to have been a fundamental mismatch between body and mind, something only correctible through social and medical transition. Changing someone's gender from male to female, or more rarely from female to male (no other alternatives were permitted), was seen as a means of last resort to help an individual otherwise unable to exist within the mainstream assume a socially viable role.

Treatment was centralized at only a few large-scale institutions, giving providers ultimate authority to determine what bodies and identities were permissible, placing their notions of trans identity ahead of our own. For some, the "born in the wrong body" narrative demanded by clinicians felt genuine; others adopted it out of desperation. But our bodies and our identities were outside our own control.

The criteria were applied with such rigidity and bias that of the two thousand people applying for gender affirming surgery at the Johns Hopkins gender clinic in its first two and a half years, only twenty-four received the procedure.[4] The other hopefuls were abandoned, unable to access care and alienated by the very professionals from whom they'd sought help.

According to the National Center for Transgender Equality (NCTE), one-third of those surveyed who received health care within the previous year reported hostility from providers, including overt verbal, physical, and sexual assault, and 23 percent did not seek care they needed out of fear.[5] Anecdotal information suggests that if we include more subtle experiences like mine above and those of individuals who did attend appointments but were not open with their providers, numbers would be far higher. Another study found that 21 percent of respondents avoided the emergency room for fear of transphobia, and that 52 percent reported negative experiences when they accessed the ER.[6]

And too many of us have suffered severe bodily trauma. Trans and gender nonbinary people are victims of intimate partner violence at rates far higher than even the rest of the LGBT community;[7] this is even more the case for trans women of color.[8] Fully half of the trans community will suffer sexual assault, and 66 percent of those attacks include other forms of sexual violence as well.[9] Trans people are similarly at risk for so-called "corrective rape"[10] or have little choice but to engage in "survival sex,"[11] again endangering our bodies and selves.

Many trans people engage in sex work, some by choice and others from need. The NCTE study mentioned above also detailed that "more than three-quarters (77%) [of trans sex workers] have experienced intimate partner violence and 72% have been sexually assaulted."

Merely growing up with an awareness of gender incongruity can be agonizing in itself. Our breasts, chests, penises, boobs, vulvae, cocks, tatas, dicks, trannyclits, cockpits, boycunts, dicklets, and lollipops are so often locations of distress that even visually acknowledging their existence can trigger anxiety, post-traumatic hyperarousal, or dissociation. Some shower in the dark, recognizing the need for proper hygiene but unable to look at physiques they find so unsettling.

We each carry these hurts and disempowerments into the treatment room. Not often enough are providers' offices places where, despite the inherent vulnerability, we feel safe.

What is the result of this antipathy, antagonism, and distrust? An adversarial therapeutic relationship yielding poor health outcomes, poorer life outcomes, and occasionally death.

Jay Kallio transitioned from female to male in 2006. Like many transgender men, it would take several years to access surgery to reshape his chest into something more masculine.

In 2008, Kallio found a lump, but after receiving a mammogram, the physician was unable to tell Kallio of the results due to his own discomfort. "In his words, he had 'a problem with [my] transgender status,' and 'I don't even know what to call you. My first thought was to send you to psychiatry' instead of removing the aggressive, HER2 positive cancer, multiplying rapidly in my chest," he later wrote. His treatment was delayed for months.

Jay ultimately passed from cancer in 2016, at age 61.

Stories like this do not build trust.

Dr. B. and all the other providers reading this: we know you want your clients to feel welcome and to get the best possible care.

We don't expect you to be experts on transgender issues. We don't need you to be experts on transgender issues.

But rather than projecting what you know, or think you know, be present with the individual in front of you. Ask what terms we prefer. Ask if you can ask about our bodies. Create an atmosphere of respect, making clear you are empathetic and honor our boundaries. Don't mention your second cousin whose child has a trans peer in class; none of us care, and it comes across as a thin attempt to claim a familiarity you haven't earned. And if it's not relevant, keep your prying to yourself. Satisfy your curiosity on the internet, like everyone else. That is what we do need.

Laura A. Jacobs, LCSW-R, is a trans- and genderqueer-identified psychotherapist, activist, author, and public speaker in the New York City area working with transgender and gender-nonbinary, LGBT, and alternate lifestyle communities of BDSM, non-monogamy, and sex work. They serve as chair of the board of directors for the Callen-Lorde Community Health Center in New York City, have been featured in television, radio, and print media, and have presented at countless community and health care conferences, professional associations, medical schools, and other organizations. Laura is the recipient of a 2018 Gay City News Impact Award, as well as the 2017 Dorothy Kartashovich Award from the Community Health Center Association of New York State. They are coauthor, with Laura Erickson-Schroth, of *"You're in the Wrong Bathroom!" and 20 Other Myths and Misconceptions about Transgender and Gender Nonconforming People*. As Lawrence Jacobs, they worked as a musician, composer, photographer, and in less glamorous corporate middle management.

Notes

1 "Trans" is used here as an umbrella term for "transgender," "genderqueer," "gender nonconforming," "gender nonbinary," and anyone who feels or expresses a gender identity other than that assigned at birth or outside the norms of society.

2 The surgeons *did* do an amazing job, but elsewhere. Buy me dinner or drinks and perhaps you will learn more.

3 Genny Beemyn, "Transgender History in the United States," in *Trans Bodies, Trans Selves: A Resource for the Transgender Community*, ed. Laura Erickson-Schroth (New York: Oxford University Press, 2014).

4 Joanne Meyerowitz, *How Sex Changed: A History of Transsexuality in the United States* (Cambridge, MA: Harvard University Press, 2002).

5 Sandy E. James, Jody L. Herman, Susan Rankin, Mara Keisling, Lisa Mottet, and Ma'ayan Anafi, *The Report of the 2015 U.S. Transgender Survey* (Washington, DC: National Center for Transgender Equality, 2016), accessed June 4, 2019, https://www.transequality.org/sites/default/files/docs/USTS-Full-Report-FINAL.PDF.

6 Greta R. Bauer, Ayden I. Scheim, Madeline B. Deutsch, and Carys Massarella, "Reported Emergency Department Avoidance, Use, and Experiences of Transgender Persons in Ontario, Canada: Results from a Respondent-Driven Sampling Survey," *Annals of Emergency Medicine* 63, no. 4 (June 2014): 713–20, accessed June 4, 2019, https://www.annemergmed.com/article/S0196-0644(13)01453-4/pdf.

7 Sabrina Gentlewarrior and Kim Fountain, *Culturally Competent Service Provision to Lesbian, Gay, Bisexual and Transgender Survivors of Sexual Violence* (Washington, DC: National Resource Center on Domestic Violence, 2009).

8 Jaime M. Grant., Lisa A. Mottet, and Justin Tanis, *Injustice at Every Turn: A Report of the National Transgender Discrimination Survey* (Washington, DC: National Center for Transgender Equality, 2011), accessed June 1, 2019, https://static1.squarespace.com/static/566c7f0c2399a3bdabb57553/t/566cbf2c57eb8de92a5392e6/1449967404768/ntds_full.pdf.

9 Office for Victims of Crime, *Responding to Transgender Victims of Sexual Assault* (Washington, DC: Office for the Victims of Crime, 2014), accessed June 4, 2019, https://www.ovc.gov/pubs/forge/.

10 "I'm going to show you what it's like to have sex with a real man" rape intended to reinforce gender norms.

11 An exchange of sex for food, shelter, or protection.

17

Tobacco-Free Queers: Prime Time to Quit

Scout

At twenty-six years old, I was one of four cochairs of what would become the largest national queer civil rights march in history. We didn't know it would be historic, we were just some of the many people who had quit their jobs and moved to DC to volunteer endless hours to keep ahead of the millions of logistical details that were part and parcel of assembling eight hundred thousand people from all fifty states.

As the months leading up to the march counted down, one big problem emerged: the National Park Service didn't want to give us a permit to march on the National Mall, the iconic home of every major civil rights march in history. All of the cochairs were young, like myself. We were all growing our connections and influence, but none of us were born into the power playing class. There was one person who reached out to us who we were hoping might be a great help, an elder LGBT statesman, friend of Hollywood elite, politicians, and major donors. We were hopeful that his connections might be able to create the kind of pressure that ultimately would get us those Mall permits from the National Park Service. But, if not that, maybe he could help secure the advance money to pay for the Jumbotron screens needed for an event this size? We eagerly agreed to meet, and when he asked to bring a reporter along, we didn't blink an eye.

We cochairs, him, and the reporter all sat down in a little café to have breakfast and discuss how his influence might be able to help the event. I hoped he would pay, because, frankly, after quitting our jobs and volunteering full-time for months, we were all living on dreams.

In all the amazing things that happened with that march, this breakfast would not be remembered as one. A month later the reporter's story came out in a national magazine. In it, we four cochairs were represented as clueless youth, well over our heads in planning such an important event. Luckily, the article implied, our elder statesman was going to be there to save the day.

I never met with him again. Despite the reporter's dismissive comments about us, the march was a huge success. The National Park Service provided the Mall permits, we secured several Jumbotrons, we even made enough money to donate the remaining funds to other nonprofits. Most importantly, people would stop us for over a decade afterwards talking about how inspirational that day was for them. How the march gave them hope of a day when LGBT people could live openly, without fear of losing their jobs or of public reprisals.

After the march I would end up defining my career in the tobacco control arena. It was here that my work overlapped again with the elder statesman, albeit with a twist. Six years after that breakfast, he was offered a consulting contract by a major tobacco company to help them win a statewide referendum threatening a large tobacco tax increase in California.[1] Industry executives knew that tobacco taxes were extremely tied to sales; it's counterintuitive but has been proven that if you want people to quit smoking, increasing the tobacco tax may well be more effective than funding cessation efforts.[2] Interestingly, documents show these executives did not want to risk being seen as targeting specific populations. So they vetoed any outreach to racial/ethnic minority communities and instead hired our elder statesman as an LGBT community expert.[3] Apparently we were one set of communities you could target with impunity.

Some of our elder statesmen's work is documented in memos forcibly disclosed by a lawsuit, memos I would discover years later when I was already running a national LGBT tobacco control network. In them I read how for 3,750 dollars per month, he assessed the situation and recommended a set of actions.[4] According to him, LGBT people were not likely supporters of the tobacco industry, but perhaps our anti-tobacco votes could be neutralized with a promotion campaign. To help the tobacco industry he made a thorough list of every LGBT media outlet in the state and painstakingly assembled the total cost of running a multimonth campaign of major ads in each outlet.[5] Sadly, the total cost of snagging the biggest ads in every single LGBT magazine and newspaper totaled probably less than a rounding error for the gargantuan tobacco industry. Since our media had a long history of being shunned by mainstream corporations who didn't want the taint of our stigma near their brands, it was inexpensive to run a large public influence campaign in our media. Face it, it still is.

What was particularly hard to swallow was how our esteemed elder statesman advised the tobacco industry to tailor their ads to us. As he relates, he wasn't able to get endorsement from our leaders but going directly to LGBT people with messages of the following issues would be compelling: lifestyle regulation, government intrusion into our private lives, and not being able to make personal choices.[6]

freedom.to speak.
to choose. to marry.
to participate. to be.
to disagree. to inhale.
to believe. to love.
to live. it's all good.
the people of santa fe natural tobacco company
No additives in our tobacco does NOT mean a safer cigarette.
SURGEON GENERAL'S WARNING: Smoking By Pregnant Women May Result in Fetal Injury, Premature Birth, And Low Birth Weight.
www.nascigs.com

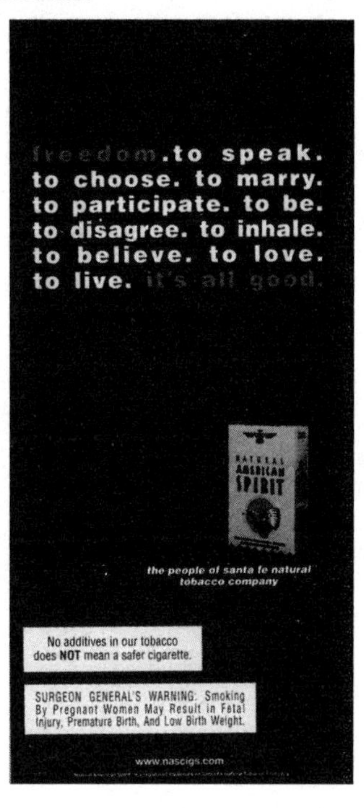

We don't have any record of what ads they placed in the long list of LGBT media outlets, but there's an ad from around that time that I suspect was informed by this advice. In it American Spirit tells customers: "Freedom, to speak, to choose, to marry . . . to inhale, to love, to live, it's all good."

Actually, it isn't all good. This ad is a perfect example of how a multinational corporation put a saddle on our civil rights battle and rode it all the way to the bank.

So is our esteemed elder statesman an anomaly? After working near the tobacco industry this long I am simply reminded of what they say about mice. If you see one, rest assured, there are dozens—if not hundreds—more behind your walls. Was he a disappointment to our communities? We all knew that he was also one of the earliest people to try and make a full-time living as an LGBT leader. That certainly wasn't easy. Many of us would go hungry trying that same gambit. Those of us who were less able to pass in mainstream culture, the brown and trans and gender variant among us, had an especially hard battle. I respect him for all that he did accomplish. I also think he was simply one in a long line of people willing to take a check without fully considering the implications to our communities' health.

This wasn't the last time I would come across signs the tobacco industry had been directly meddling with our opinions and leadership. That same Master Settlement Agreement that created the tobacco industry documents library also forced the tobacco industry to provide funding for an independent national foundation dedicated to tobacco control. This foundation, the Truth Initiative, has created some of the most compelling ads we had ever seen about avoiding tobacco use. I was delighted one day when Cheryl Healton, the then executive director of the foundation, came over and told me they had finally decided to make an ad that specifically focused on queers. In particular, they were highlighting another old tobacco industry marketing document, one that was labeled "Project SCUM". While SCUM stood for Sub Culture Urban Marketing, the ad campaign was actually aimed at homeless people and gay men.[7] Ironically a few years later the same company was placing an ad in LGBT community event programs that stated: "Whenever someone yells 'Dude that's so gay.' We'll be there."[8] Apparently their private and public opinion of us differed.

I was extremely happy to hear Truth was finally doing a queer ad. I shouldn't have been so happy so fast. The reason Cheryl came to talk to me was because two-thirds of the television stations they wanted to run the ad on weren't willing to run it, because . . . well, queer. I was very upset and immediately realized I needed to connect Truth with GLAAD, our national group that works to ensure media representations of us are fair and nondiscriminatory. But then my shoulders slumped—big tobacco had gotten there first. Lucky Strike was in the middle of years of being a corporate sponsor of GLAAD's black-tie galas.[9] We had already tried to strategize about how to encourage GLAAD to refuse their funding. A friend of mine even made a very amusing video about this sponsorship, *How They Get Us to Screw Ourselves*, and showed it at queer film festivals across the country.[10] So here we were standing on the threshold of our biggest media spotlight ever to the problem of LGBT smoking, and thanks to a little careful sponsorship, we were not able to fight back against the old-school discrimination that was keeping our ad off the air. GLAAD wasn't so unusual for that time; other organizations were also taking tobacco industry ads. Many, like GLAAD, have now stopped.

Later years were aswirl with shadows and rumors about tobacco industry activities in queer communities around the country.

Community bars in different cities reported they were contractually unable to host any tobacco control activities. A self-claimed LGBT business owner spoke out against clean indoor air in St. Louis, but when we researched him, we couldn't find any business he owned, and the same person had protested clean indoor air laws states away as well. Was he a fabrication of the tobacco industry? Reports of that trend continued: my own home state of Rhode Island delayed full adoption of clean indoor air laws, because the LGBT bar owners protested they would get disproportionately hurt by the new laws; clean indoor air laws in DC and Georgia also met opposition from LGBT community leaders. Did this opposition represent our community opinion? Quite the opposite. Like the esteemed elder statesman had noted, we were not naturally supporters of the tobacco industry. A contemporaneous Harris Interactive nationwide poll showed LGBT people actually were more willing than others to pay extra for a smoke-free bar.[11] After we got a small grant from Robert Wood Johnson Foundation, I got to work closely around this phenomena in DC.

It quickly became apparent how this game worked. The tobacco industry would recruit some LGBT leader, usually a nightlife promoter or bar owner, then this contractee would start to speak up about the negative impact of clean indoor air laws on LGBT people in particular. Legislators, reasonably wary of further upsetting the activist heavy LGBT civil rights fighters, would then back off and make clean indoor air concessions. Until we got our grant rolling in DC that same pattern was happening there. A big nightlife promoter kept publishing articles about the negative impact of clean indoor air laws. When we came in and provided a countering voice, leaders jumped on with us, and eventually the LGBT communities were actually acknowledged as key in passing clean indoor air legislation. But in most states, when the tobacco industry moved in to recruit one of our community leaders, there was no opposition. It was a very effective tactic.

How many times was this tactic used to derail clean indoor air efforts? I heard about four times. I wonder how many mice were in that house? And don't even get me started on the rumor of a Pride director of a fine southern state who was offered the car of his choice, if he simply accepted tobacco underwriting for Pride. Did this really happen? The tobacco industry is no longer compelled to disclose documents, so we will certainly never know. For years, we would approach community magazines about not taking tobacco ads, and even after other advertisers opened their purse strings publishers would tell us bald-facedly: "We have to take these ads or we will close." Don't think these ads don't drive editorial coverage too. Analyses of our community media show that even the editorial coverage is overwhelmingly likely to be pro-tobacco or at least neutral.[12] Because we have been ignored by so many, because we have suffered such stigma, and in part because other people do not want to upset us, we have unwittingly been pawns for the tobacco industry to deploy in their larger legislative battles.

We've been pawns for the tobacco industry. So what? Tobacco companies were one of the few willing to support us early on; we are grateful for that. There are actually focus groups showing that while other communities were upset about this targeting, we were grateful.[13] Again, it just shows how far along we are developmentally as a set of communities. But back to my point: So what?

Sadly, just as much attention as the tobacco industry has paid us, the tobacco control arena has not. Let's take one simple example. Stop right now and ask yourself, "What is the largest health risk is for the LGBT communities?" If you're anything like the general population or the thousands of LGBT people surveyed over the years, you will say things like: HIV, mental health, suicide. In fact, on average, tobacco use is only listed as the ninth or tenth top health concern. But epidemiologically it affects about six times as many of us as are HIV positive, and most of those affected will lose years off their life due to tobacco use. In other words, by the numbers, tobacco use is the single largest LGBT health threat, by far. We use tobacco products at rates over 40 percent higher than the general population.[14] But the truth is most of us don't even realize we have a smoking disparity, much less that it's our single top health threat. Now think of this, how many LGBT-tailored tobacco cessation programs have you seen? How many LGBT-tailored HIV programs have you seen? We only wish the tobacco control funders would treat us as well as the tobacco industry does.

The impact in years lost from our communities is only one part of the picture. We once worked with Centers for Disease Control and Prevention (CDC) epidemiologists to help us calculate the total cost of queer tobacco use in dollars. Even back in 2014, how much were we as a set of communities spending on cigarettes each year in the U.S. alone? By all available data, the best estimate is 7.9 billion dollars a year.[15] Yes, that's a "b." Think of where we'd be if even a fraction of that money stayed in our communities, instead of being siphoned off to line the pockets of a set of multinational corporations.

Now the game is shifting; youth are being lured into tobacco addiction through vaping. Many mistakenly think vaping products do not contain addictive nicotine. Even if they know these products do contain nicotine, the lure of candy flavorings, a glowing electronic delivery device, and the promise of "healthier" tobacco consumption are proving too hard to ignore. In public health terms, where populations tend to adopt new behaviors slowly, the number of youth vaping is going through the roof. We are seeing faster adoption of this new nicotine delivery device than practically any other public health risk on record. And, of course, like with cigarettes, LGBT youth are vaping at much higher rates than others. Are we being specially targeted? Imagine me shrugging. I doubt this house is mouse-free yet. Even if the tobacco industry isn't reaching out to give us any special attention, we are already made vulnerable by the stigma and discrimination we experience in the world at large. Starting smoking or vaping is mostly a young person's sport, few pick this habit up after they turn twenty. So as long as the queer youth suicide rate stays high, it seems extremely likely that we will turn to risky stress relievers as part of our efforts to cope.

We may be smoking at higher rates than others, we may hand over huge pots of cash to the tobacco industry, we may not realize how we've been targeted and manipulated by them, but there is great movement afoot to change the tide. We are seeing a steady uptick in the number of states that are funding LGBT-tailored tobacco control programs; for example, the editor of this book runs just such a statewide tobacco control program. We are also seeing more targeted media campaigns. We are seeing an increased interest in making sure tobacco quitlines are queer-welcoming. So much so that it's highly likely when you call 1-800-QUIT-NOW, you will reach a quitline that's had specific training on how to be welcoming. We have also seen the biggest ever federal LGBT health initiative roll out in the United States, This Free Life, a thirty-five-million-dollar multiyear project aimed at reducing queer smoking disparities.[16] You can go on the federal homepage for that project and see dozens of edgy real-people ads talking about the power of saying no to tobacco. The CDC has been funding the LGBT tobacco disparity network I run for over a dozen years, and slowly we are making inroads in both educating queer leadership about the impact tobacco has on our communities and educating tobacco control programs about the need to tailor their work to us.

As a result of all this work, we are seeing a downward trend in our own community smoking rates. The downturn is not as fast as with the general population, but it is heading in the right direction. Most importantly, every day dozens of queer people across the U.S. are starting their quit attempts. It still usually takes many tries to be wholly successful, but every step along that journey brings all of us closer to freedom.

I went to an amazing memorial service for a hugely loved man, Chris Harris. To celebrate his life, his people rented out the whole top floor ballroom of the grandest hotel in town. Several drag queens performed, and his loved ones spoke tearfully about how much energy he'd brought into the local community. Then we gathered downstairs as a local brass band played. We decorated ourselves with rainbow flags, light-up sticks, and glitter, then hundreds of us trooped into the street where the police motorcycles and band led our fine parade across town to the second half of the party, with dancing and more performances that would continue into the night. As we walked I saw his picture in lights on the forty-foot tall sign for our performing arts center. After news of his death spread, he was quickly named honorary chair of Pride in both Providence and Boston. Here was a man who was an icon in his community. Like many of us, his voice was silenced much too early. In his case it was literally silenced, he was a Rhode Island LGBT bar owner and promoter who had long ago had his voice box removed as a result of his laryngeal cancer. While some bar owner in this state was once recruited by the tobacco industry to speak up against clean indoor air, I prefer the words of this bar owner. As relayed by one of the people speaking at his memorial service: "Don't smoke."

Scout is the deputy director of the National LGBT Cancer Project and the principal investigator of the CDC-funded LGBT tobacco-related cancer disparity network. In this capacity he spends much of his time providing technical assistance for governmental tobacco and cancer focusing agencies, expanding their reach and engagement with LGBT populations. He leads a team of specialists in the Rhode Island office who focus especially on building tools and sharing strategies across state departments of health. Scout is also an expert cultural competency trainer and sought after public speaker. He has a long history in health policy analysis and a particular interest in expanding LGBT surveillance and research. He is a member of the NIH Council of Councils and the chair of the NIH Sexual and Gender Minority Work Group. His work has won him recognition from the U.S. House of Representatives, two state governments, and many city governments. Scout is an openly transgender father of three, a vegetarian, and an avid hiker.

Notes

1 "May 28 Industry Meeting—CA Initiative," RJ Reynolds Records, June 1, 1968, accessed June 4, 2019, https://www.industrydocumentslibrary.ucsf.edu/tobacco/docs/zrfb0054.

2 Frank Chaloupka, Kurt Straif, and Maria E. Leon, "Effectiveness of Tax and Price Policies in Tobacco Control," *Tobacco Control* 20, no. 3 (May 2011), accessed June 4, 2019, https://hal.archives-ouvertes.fr/hal-00589445/document.

3 "May 28 Industry Meeting."

4 "Corporate Affairs 990000 Original Budget," Philip Morris Records, October 10, 1998, accessed June 4, 2019, https://www.industrydocumentslibrary.ucsf.edu/tobacco/docs/nxnv0226.

5 David Mixner to Grant Gillham, "Subject: Report," Tobacco Institute Records, June 9, 1998; RPCI Tobacco Institute and Council for Tobacco Research Records.

6 Ibid.

7 Joel P. Engardio, "Smoking Gun—Tobacco Industry Documents Expose an R.J. Reynolds Marketing Plan Targeting S.F. Gays and Homeless People. Its Name: Project SCUM," *SF Weekly*, May 2, 2001, accessed June 4, 2019, https://archives.sfweekly.com/sanfrancisco/smoking-gun/Content?oid=2141586.

8 Fizza Imran, "LGBT History Month: How Has Tobacco Advertising Affected Health Disparities?" Suwannee River Area Health Education Center, October 31, 2017, accessed June 4, 2019. https://srahec.org/lgbt-history-month-tobacco-advertising/.

9 Perry Stevens, Lisa M. Carlson, and Johanna M. Hinman, "An Analysis of Tobacco Industry Marketing to Lesbian, Gay, Bisexual, and Transgender (LGBT) Populations: Strategies for Mainstream Tobacco Control and Prevention," *Health Promotion Practice* 5, no. 3, supplement (July 2004): S129–S134, accessed June 4, 2019, http://citeseerx.ist.psu.edu/viewdoc/download?doi=10.1.1.865.5083&rep=rep1&type=pdf.

10 Bob Gordon, *How They Get Us to Screw Ourselves*, accessed June 4, 2019, https://www.youtube.com/watch?v=F5-6eH18E4U.

11 "Six Out of Ten Adults Surveyed Prefer Smoke-Free Bars and Clubs," Harris Interactive, accessed May 23, 2005, unavailable June 4, 2019, http://www.harrisinteractive.com/news/allnewsbydate.asp?NewsID=566.

12 Elizabeth A. Smith, Naphtali Offen, and Ruth E. Malone, "Pictures Worth a Thousand Words: Noncommercial Tobacco Content in the Lesbian, Gay, and Bisexual Press," *Journal of Health Communication* 11, no. 7 (October–November 2006), accessed June 4, 2019, https://www.ncbi.nlm.nih.gov/pmc/articles/PMC2836900/.

13 Elizabeth A. Smith, Katherine Thomson, Naphtali Offen, and Ruth E. Malone, "'If You Know You Exist, It's Just Marketing Poison': Meanings of Tobacco Industry Targeting in the Lesbian, Gay, Bisexual, and Transgender Community," *American Journal of Public Health* 98, no. 6 (June 2008): 996–1003, accessed June 4, 2019, https://www.ncbi.nlm.nih.gov/pmc/articles/PMC2377293/.

14 Teresa W. Wang, Kat Asman, Andrea S. Gentzke, Karen A. Cullen, Enver Holder-Hayes, Carolyn Reyes-Guzman, Ahmed Jamal, Linda Neff, and Brian A. King, "Tobacco Product Use Among Adults—United States, 2017," *Morbidity and Mortality Weekly Report* 67, no. 44 (November 9, 2018): 1225–32, accessed June 4, 2019, https://www.cdc.gov/mmwr/volumes/67/wr/mm6744a2.htm; Francisco O. Buchting, Kristen E. Emory, Scout, Yoonsang Kim, Pebbles Fagan, Lisa E. Vera, and Sherry Emery, "Transgender Use of Cigarettes, Cigars, and E-Cigarettes in a National Study," *American Journal of Preventive Medicine* 53, no. 1 (July 2017): e1-e7.

15 "LGBT Tobacco Infograph Citations," LGBT Health Link, January 16, 2014, accessed June 4, 2019, https://blog.lgbthealthlink.org/2014/01/16/tobacco-infograph-citations/.

16 "Pick Your Poison," This Free Life, accessed June 4, 2019, https://thisfreelife.betobaccofree.hhs.gov/pick-your-poison.

18

Challenging HIV Stigma

Sean Strub

Biomedical advances against HIV since the dawn of the epidemic have been nothing short of astonishing. An almost always fatal disease is now, for those with the privilege of access to treatment, a manageable chronic illness, treated with a single daily pill. A person who acquires HIV today has every reason to expect to live a normal lifespan.

Yet with such astonishing success in treatment, why is HIV stigma worse today than ever before? Why do so many long-term survivors, including many who were exceptionally open about their HIV positive status for years, find they must now keep it a secret, sometimes going deeply into closets they thought they had left for good years ago?

Many people—especially those who do not have HIV—find these questions startling. That's because they remember the days when one had to wear a spacesuit to visit a person with AIDS in a hospital or was afraid to eat in a restaurant with gay waiters or refused to touch a person they thought might have the virus.

Those are all stigmatizing reactions—born of combinations of fear, ignorance, and bias—but they are ultimately about fear of casual contagion. Today we know so much more about the real routes and risks of HIV transmission, as evidenced by surveys showing the number of people who believe they can get HIV from a drinking glass or sitting on a toilet seat has dropped dramatically.

But to the stigmatized person, the person living with HIV (PLHIV), the stigma is far more nuanced and complex than simple fear of casual contagion. The stigma is about our moral worth being judged when others find out we have the virus. It is about our words being discounted before they leave our mouths, marginalization, "othering," and, very importantly, self-stigmatization and the internalized stigma we absorb from the broader society.

By those measures, many long-term survivors agree that the stigma has worsened. Unfortunately, there is no pill to cure stigma, but it can be lessened with a better understanding of where it comes from and how best to address it.

In the early years of the epidemic, most people who had moral or religious concerns with homosexuality, promiscuity, sex work, or drug use, saw PLHIV through a "hate the sin, love the sinner" type of pseudo-sympathetic lens. We were in pain, suffering, at times looked grotesque, and were expected to die, probably very soon and possibly in a horrific manner.

In the mid-nineties, combination therapy was introduced, and the broader society began to understand that we were no longer dying, but, in fact, we were going to live. Instead of being seen through the lens of our likely demise, we were seen through the lens of our potential survival. If we were living longer, it meant we would be around longer to potentially transmit HIV to others.

The public health and criminal justice systems began to consider us as an inherently dangerous population and a threat to society. We became seen as people who needed to be tracked down, identified, tested, listed, reported, regulated, and, increasingly, criminalized. Those with deep-seated bias against the populations at greatest risk of acquiring HIV felt like a renewed license to demonize us.

The media played a role as well. In those early years, there was a steady flow of feature coverage in the media, inspiring stories about the triumph of the human spirit. The woman working two jobs and raising children, even while managing a serious life-threatening illness. The child born with HIV who valiantly struggles to go to school and be like the other kids. The two men with AIDS who took care of each other, bringing joy to their final months, weeks, and days.

That kind of media coverage has largely disappeared. Today, when a person with HIV is mentioned by name in a media context, it is frequently in a criminal context: an "HIV predator," "AIDS monster," or burdened with similarly pejorative labels in sensationalized, if not hysterical, coverage.

Beyond the public health and criminal justice systems and the media, another factor is how the importance of connecting people living with HIV with each other, once considered absolutely critical, has been downgraded, ignored, and with many service providers is no longer seen as a priority.

In the early years, unless a person was in an acute medical crisis at the time of their diagnosis, the most important post-diagnosis priority was to get the person together with others living with HIV, through a support group, PLHIV network, or other mechanism.

Connecting with others enabled us to ask questions, educate ourselves, and build a network of support to enable us to deal with the consequences of HIV, including disclosing that we have it to our sexual partners, friends, family, and coworkers. It was through these support groups and networks that PLHIV became empowered advocates, for ourselves, each other, and our community.

Hundreds of HIV service providers, including major agencies such as Gay Men's Health Crisis (GMHC), San Francisco AIDS Foundation, AIDS Project Los Angeles, and others, were founded by people with AIDS, our partners, and our closest friends, including many who didn't know at the time if they had the virus or not.

The existing health care service delivery structure couldn't serve us, didn't want to serve us, which necessitated our creation of a parallel network on a peer-to-peer service delivery model. There were no meetings of boards of directors where members of those boards referred to the agency's clients as "them," because clients were in the room, sitting on the board, and serving on the staff. We were not just at the table, we helped decide who else would be at the table.

Over time, as the epidemic grew and service providers "professionalized," they also began to incrementally move away from the peer-to-peer service delivery model we pioneered, toward the more dominant "benefactor-victim" model, where self-empowerment ideals are not as important.

Those boards of directors that were once all or nearly all people living with HIV transformed into boards where there was no, little, or only token PLHIV representation on them. Funding for support groups and networks was reduced or eliminated. The concept of connecting the newly diagnosed with other PLHIV became a quaint relic from the past, in favor of a mistaken belief that we would treat our way out of the epidemic.

Today the top priority after a person is diagnosed is, typically, to get that person on anti-retroviral treatment, so they will not pose a risk of

HIV transmission to others. There are vastly fewer support groups and networks, and referrals to them are a rare exception, no longer the rule.

Today when a newly diagnosed person is given this life-changing news, they are put on treatment, told to come back in three months, and ejected onto the sidewalk, expected to go about their lives as if it was no big deal. Yet HIV stigma makes many of us reluctant to share this news with our friends and families. We keep it a secret out of shame, fear, or a preference for keeping our personal health information private.

Shame because most everyone knows how not to acquire HIV today, unlike the "innocent" seroconversions of years past, and we live in a culture of blame. When a person is diagnosed, they are subject to harsh judgment, including from many in the communities that a few years ago were the beacons of hope and bastions of support.

Fear also encourages secrecy about one's HIV positive status. Years ago, when a diagnosis meant a person was probably going to become ill, we didn't worry as much about who knew we had HIV or our long-term career prospects. Our survival timeline and focus were much shorter.

Today, a person with HIV may understandably want to avoid becoming defined by their condition, being subject to the gossip of coworkers, or having their HIV status become an impediment to career advancement. They have the choice of keeping their diagnosis a secret, living a normal lifespan, and are not likely to show evidence of HIV through wasting, visible Kaposi's Sarcoma lesions, or other indices.

It is, after all, private information, no one else's business, so keeping one's HIV positive diagnosis a secret is an important right that every person with HIV should enjoy, if they choose. But it also can contribute to isolation, self-stigmatization, and rendering the epidemic less present and less visible to others.

The community context associated with disclosure of one's HIV status is also different. Once the LGBT community accepted the epidemic as a collective responsibility, wrapping its arms around those newly diagnosed, expressing its love and support, and sending a message, "We'll get through this together." Such is no longer the case, as the LGBT movement moved on to marriage equality, military service, and other priorities.

Even within gay men's social sexual circles it is very different, with the online hookup apps full of guys who assert they are "clean" and running away from those who bravely share their HIV positive status. Instead of getting love and support, many gay men with HIV are made to feel like pariahs, as though they don't deserve as satisfying and fulfilling intimate life as everyone else.

The reality is that the consequences of disclosure are greater today than they were years ago. If we want to encourage PLHIV to disclose, then we must prioritize making it safer to disclose, not wagging fingers at us telling us what we "should" do. Making it safer to disclose means combating stigma.

Anti-stigma efforts have typically focused almost exclusively on settings where stigma occurs (places of employment, in the health care and educational systems) and on trying to "educate" the stigmatizers. The stigmatized—those of us living with HIV—were sitting on the sidelines, waiting to benefit from the enlightenment thus resulting.

Yet a far more effective strategy to reduce stigma is found by focusing on empowering the stigmatized, rather than educating the stigmatizers. The Civil Rights Movement in the 1960s didn't gain traction and make progress because a white supremacist majority woke up one day and got educated and decided not to be racist; it made progress because a black minority became empowered, outspoken, and demanded equity.

"Empowerment" has become a buzzword to the extent that it is practically like white noise, having lost any real meaning. Years ago, the U.S. Supreme Court Justice Potter Stewart, in a decision defining what was pornographic, noted he had a hard time defining it but said, "I know it when I see it." That's a bit how I feel about the empowerment of PLHIV.

Empowerment isn't something that one individual or agency can give to another; it is something that arises organically when the conditions are right. Those conditions start with creating opportunities for people living with HIV to connect with each other, whether for social or peer support, for recreation, or to pursue advocacy or educational agendas.

Michael Callen, one of the first AIDS activists, used to say that there was "a special magic" when there were only people living with HIV or AIDS in the room. The conversation is different when stigmatized individuals are able to be with each other, free of the judgment and stigma they typically experience in their lives. In those spaces, we are able to discuss and share our concerns and priorities in a more gentle and generous way, free of polarizing interests that want us to fit their agendas.

When people living with HIV are able to get together, they then have the opportunity to create their own agenda, select leadership that can be held accountable to other PLHIV and, importantly, speak with a collective voice. People living with HIV who are connected with other PLHIV, through support groups, PLHIV networks, or other means, report much higher self-empowerment, are better able to handle stigma, and have a better quality of life and improved health outcomes.

Peer support is vital for every person in every phase of their lives, to be sure. But the more disenfranchised, marginalized, or stigmatized the community, the more important it is. For those of us lucky enough to have survived the epidemic so far—in many cases having come to the brink of death before returning, Lazarus-like, to a bonus round of life we never expected to see—finding support from each other is more important than ever.

Sean Strub is a longtime activist and writer who has been HIV positive for more than thirty-three years. He is the founder of *POZ* magazine, the leading independent global source of information about HIV, and served as its publisher and executive editor from 1994 to 2004. He presently serves as the executive director of the Sero Project, a network of people with HIV fighting for freedom from stigma and injustice. Strub was active with the People with AIDS Coalition/New York in the mid-eighties, cochaired the fundraising committee for ACT UP/New York in the late eighties, and in 1990 became the first openly HIV positive person to run for the U.S. Congress. He is the author of *Body Counts: A Memoir of Politics, Sex, AIDS, and Survival.*

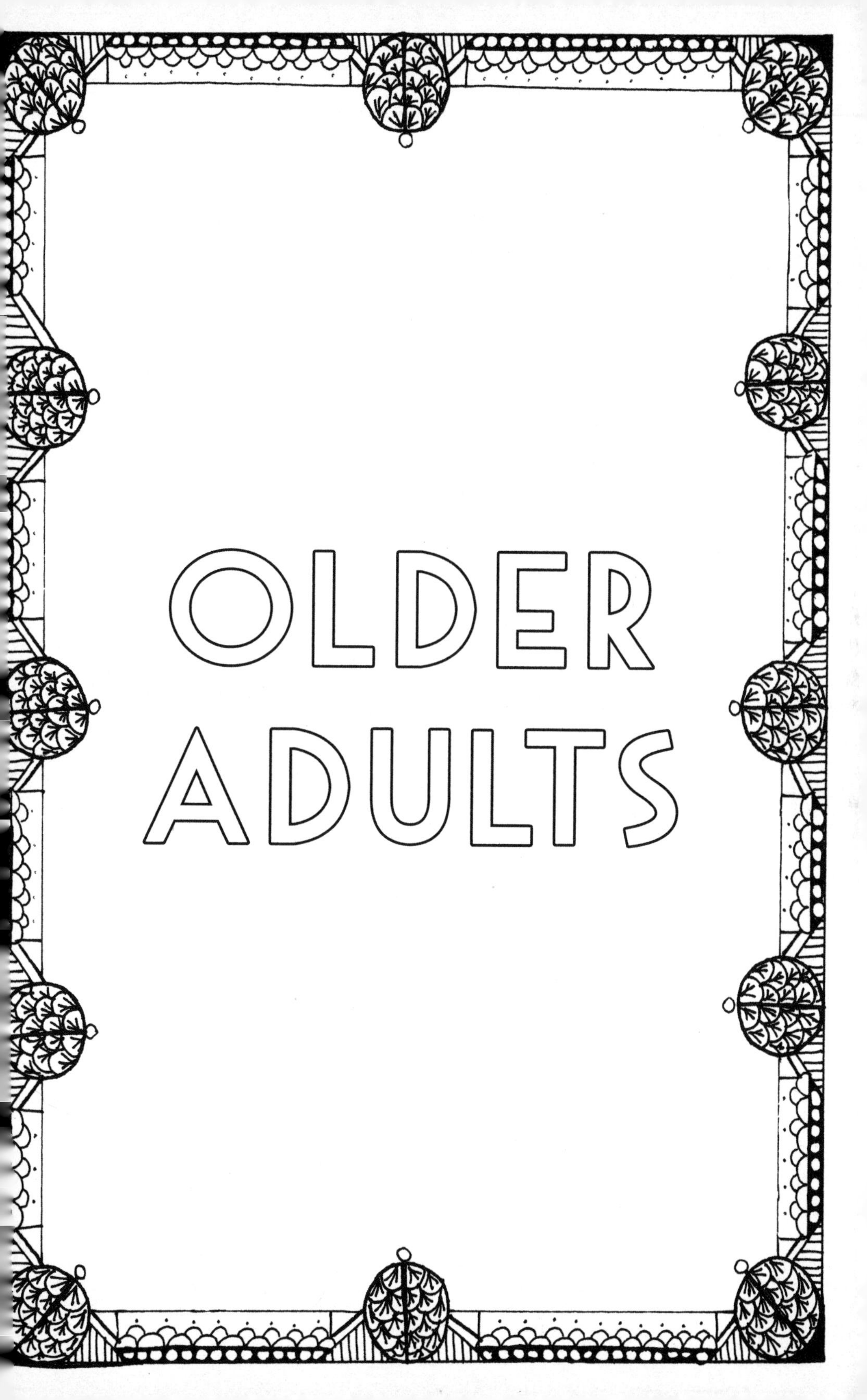

OLDER ADULTS

19

Archiving AIDS: Intergenerational Education About an Epidemic

Chris Bartlett

In 1990, I was twenty-four years old and in the midst of a crisis. I had returned to Philadelphia after three years abroad, and my community was facing its biggest challenge to date: the emergence of HIV within all generations of gay men. Many of my friends had died, and I had become caretaker to a few. I began showing up at Monday night meetings at ACT UP Philadelphia at the cozy Church of Saint Luke and the Epiphany on 13th Street.

This was five years before the emergence of the protease inhibitors that would make HIV a chronic manageable disease for those who could access medications. Many of the men on the floor of the ACT UP meetings were living with HIV, and some of them were very sick. There was a sense of urgency in the room—that we could and would do anything to save another life.

In those Monday night meetings, I met many lions of the HIV activist movement, including Kiyoshi Kuromiya, Jonathan Lax, Lois Lax, Anna Forbes, and Dominic Bash. Each of these activists in their own way taught me strategies for impacting social change and surviving for the long term as a person committed to moving the ball forward on the key issues of the day.

Importantly, these activists were a generation older than I was and had experienced other activist movements. They brought with them to our Monday night meetings their experience and strength from having participated in these efforts. I paid attention to these predecessors, and did my best to learn from their example.

For instance, Kiyoshi had built bridges between what was then called Gay Liberation and numerous other social movements. He had been friends with Martin Luther King, organized LGBT workshops at Black Panther national congresses, organized a famous demonstration at University of Pennsylvania that brought thousands of people onto the campus to protest the Vietnam War, and, when I knew him, successfully organized a lawsuit at the Supreme Court to ensure that the internet would not be censored from providing lifesaving safer-sex or other health-related information. His lawsuit was victorious.

Kiyoshi, through his example, showed us the power of what would now be called intersectionality. In those days, we called it liberation. But this was the idea that our activist efforts would be strengthened by working alongside and within other movements. In ACT UP Philadelphia, we provided clinic defense to Planned Parenthood. We showed up at the jails to advocate for prisoners with AIDS. We raided the school board to give the superintendent an "F" for her inaction on condoms in the schools. Kiyoshi showed us that we were strengthened by our solidarity with each other.

One key strategy for health promotion, I've found, is to root one's health practice in the context of a multigenerational effort, such as the one I participated in with ACT UP Philadelphia. By this I mean, the strategies we implement to pursue community health in the present are connected to many generations of work by our activist elders and ancestors from the past.

I was well-trained by my mentor Eric Rofes, the well-known LGBT health theorist, to root theory and practice in efforts that had come before. Rofes, who was part of the first generation of LGBT liberation activists, published his community organizing ideas in the seminal *Gay Community News*. He then implemented those ideas in his work in LGBT community centers and AIDS service organizations and helped to create models that became part of efforts to support people living with AIDS, their caregivers, and a whole generation of LGBT people who, though not infected, were deeply impacted by the epidemic.

Rofes always credited the historical movements that came before: he acknowledged the lessons of the women's health movement and its seminal work, *Our Bodies, Our Selves* (1970). He celebrated the history of black medical clinics created by black communities for black communities. And he showed how health organizing underpinned many of the social change movements of the sixties. He also taught me to include the leaders of these movements in our own so that their wisdom and skills could be put to bear on our own work.

Grounding our health promotion work in movement history helps us to understand our hard work in organizing as part of an effort that goes back decades and that will continue into the future long after we are gone.

I have also looked to Jewish practice for inspiration over the years. I have been struck by the Jewish reverence for life, even after people have died. While reading stories of the Holocaust, I was impressed by the fact that Jews who had survived the Nazi genocide were committed to making sure that not one Jew who was murdered would be forgotten or undocumented. For each European city, town, or village whose Jews who had been murdered, scholars took the time to document every name, every family. Hundreds of volumes of books were completed detailing these lives and providing a portrait of the Jewish culture and community in these localities at the time of the Holocaust.

I was struck by this dedication to memory, history, and life. Holocaust survivors recognized that to forget the lives of these ancestors was to forget the powerful stories of their lives and the roles that they played in the community fabric. Remembering them through the process of cataloging their names had the benefit of countering the erasure of their history by the Nazis. It also inspired future generations to live their lives with generational remembrance and resilience.

I began to think about my own relationship to dozens of friends who had died of AIDS during the pretreatment years of the AIDS epidemic (roughly 1981–1995). I knew many powerful activists who had fought to find a cure for AIDS within their own lives. Many of these activists had been architects of the LGBT movement and many other political movements—and I wanted to make sure that their stories were preserved in a place where they could easily be referenced. Further, I wanted to commit to the possibility that their stories could be steadily updated by any contributor. I wanted to create a Wiki to catalogue all of the gay men who had died of AIDS in Philadelphia.

I started by reaching out to the Philadelphia Department of Health to find out what I didn't know. How many gay men had died since 1981? I was told that 4,600 men had died. That was a staggering number for me—and I knew that a loss of that many people from our community must have had a tremendous impact physically, emotionally, and spiritually.

The William Way LGBT Community Center in Philadelphia is home to the John J. Wilcox, Jr. Archives, one of the largest LGBT-specific archives in the U.S. More than forty years of collecting have yielded the stories of our communities' members from many organizations, social groups, bars, and events. I'm thrilled that the archives play a role in assisting new generations of activists to understand their connection to the movements that inspired their own work and that can teach new generations of LGBT people about the history of AIDS and the memories those of us who lived through it hold.

In 2018, we worked on a powerful exhibit that is a great example—the story of the Mariel Boatlift and the LGBT Marielitos who arrived in Philadelphia. This story too is intergenerational and shows the threads of activism through decades. In June 1980, Cuba allowed a wave of emigrants to come to the United States. President Jimmy Carter arranged for the immigrants to be transported to settlement camps, including one at Fort Indiantown Gap, Pennsylvania. Among these immigrants, the so-called Marielitos, were many LGBT individuals.

In one of the first acts of national LGBT political organizing, the Metropolitan Community Church (MCC)—an LGBT denomination—organized Spanish-speaking volunteers to visit Fort Indiantown Gap and the other settlement camps to arrange permanent housing for these immigrants. From Philadelphia, longtime activists Ada Bello and John Cunningham, as well as *Philadelphia Gay News* reporter Mark Segal, traveled to Fort Indiantown Gap to meet with Marielitos and to help connect them to host homes.

Through the work of these activists and others, hundreds of Marielitos were settled in LGBT or LGBT-friendly households to smooth their entry into the U.S. and their path to citizenship. I was inspired by this story, both because it was an early example of pre-AIDS national organizing and because it showed LGBT people stepping outside of their natural political arena to support those from a different country with a different language who had urgent needs in their communities. The voices of the activists who supported the Marielitos remind us of the importance of supporting the many undocumented immigrants who are now threatened by immigration policies of the U.S. today.

While organizing the Marielito archives exhibit at William Way, we were again reminded of the impact of AIDS on so many generations. The Cuban immigrants had arrived in 1980, and AIDS was identified in the media in June of 1981. Many of the Cuban immigrants, freed from homophobic oppression in Cuba, dove with gusto into the liberated sexual life of American cities. Many were infected with HIV, and many died. But the activists who had worked to support the immigrants maintained contact with those who survived, and we were able to find pictures and stories of the ones who had passed at such a young age. Images from the Fort Indiantown Gap settlement center show a joyous crew of young LGBT folks awaiting their host homes.

As the exhibit came close to being mounted, I received a call from a lesbian who had been actively involved in the early organizing to support the Marielitos. She told me that she had recently reconnected with one of the refugees, now in his sixties, who had told her about the William Way exhibit and credited her activism with giving him hope and saving his life. Both the activist and the man she had helped attended the exhibit opening, engaging with other people who had participated in this important historical event.

When I think back over twenty-five years of LGBT activism, I wonder how, without these archives, new generations of LGBT people would learn about our community's history of fighting for equitable treatment from the government, organizations, and pharmaceutical companies when so many of us were dying from AIDS. The LGBT community is one in which we often grow up without families who share our identities—we don't learn the stories and histories of our culture from our parents. We need to learn it from each other.

Just as Jewish activists have gone to great length to document, preserve, and educate new generations of Jewish people about the Holocaust, so they can say, "Never again!" so too must be the case for LGBT activists. When we remember, we can fight back against current bias, we can insist that the government care about LGBT health. We can ensure that drugs are available and affordable to provide the care we need. And we can call out institutions that don't provide culturally appropriate care.

When we actively remember the pain of the past, we can build resiliency for a healthier future.

Chris Bartlett is the executive director of the William Way Lesbian, Gay, Bisexual and Transgender (LGBT) Community Center in Philadelphia. For more than twenty-five years, he has been an innovative thinker and leader in technology-driven community organizing, having led the SafeGuards Gay Men's Health Project, the LGBT Community Assessment, and the national LGBT Leadership Initiative. He serves on the LGBT commissions for both the City of Philadelphia and the Commonwealth of Pennsylvania.

20

Organizing against Social Isolation: Older Lesbians in Rural Communities

Kat Carrick and Ntlotleng Mabena

Social isolation has been linked in several studies to poor health outcomes. While social isolation can be difficult to navigate for many throughout their lifespan, in the LGBT community, it can be particularly challenging for older lesbians in rural communities.

As coauthors, we have a history of lesbian community activism. For more than thirty years now, Kat has organized lesbian social events, Parents and Friends of Lesbians and Gays (PFLAG) groups,[1] and served as a "staff syster" at many women's festivals. She has also served as volunteer, board member, grant writer, and cochair of the Gay and Lesbian Community Center of Pittsburgh (now operating as the Pittsburgh Equality Center). Coming of age as a baby dykling during the early years of the AIDS epidemic galvanized her commitment to crafting community events. Her frequent moves throughout the United States provided opportunities to hone her community organizing skills in urban, suburban, and rural areas.

Ntlotleng is a public health clinician working with black lesbians in the Gauteng Townships in South Africa. Although not considered rural, townships are areas where many live in adversity and poverty, with limited access to resources. She has provided HIV care and safe abortion services, linked many to substance use treatment and support services, and provided post-rape care to lesbians from these specific communities. Her passion lies in working with marginalized women and making sure that all women, especially the most vulnerable, have access to quality primary health care services.

While it has been astounding to witness the speed of advancement for LGBT human rights in our world in recent years, many benefits have yet to be fully realized in rural communities. The LGBT community owes a debt of gratitude for the individuals who literally put their lives on the line. Yet, even in the United States, LGBT legal protections against discrimination and rights procured through legislative changes remain precarious and under threat of obliteration by executive order. And internationally, human rights and health for LGBT people varies widely from country to country, with hostile laws contributing significantly to negative health impacts.

Often those most vulnerable to social stigma and discrimination live in the margins of our world. Navigating heteronormative social expectations and cultural intersections can be challenging for many in the LGBT community, but the intersections of older-age, lesbian identity, and rural geography can lead to social isolation. Living in isolated rural communities, challenges may include invisibility or denial of significant relationships. One rural lesbian, graduating with her master's degree, coped with the stress of having to explain her partner by introducing her as "my friend who agreed to take pictures for me." The erasure of not having her partner recognized as family was palpable when she was surrounded by classmates taking family photos. Considerable emotional expenditure is required to maintain the illusion of being single when partnered, to come to terms with identity and labels, and to engage in daily decisions about coming out to others, given the potential ramifications.

In rural communities, each interaction occurs within a social context defined by isolation and limited support or exposure to positive LGBT role models. Rural life can necessitate consideration of immediate and lifelong consequences of roles and of acceptance by community members. Each interaction in rural communities can be a potential risk to social capital (by family, friends, or spiritual communities), risk of financial security (threat to employment or housing), risk to custody or visitation with children, risk of violence (hate crimes), or risk of ill-treatment if dependent on caregivers. This chapter will address these risk factors and discuss strategies to strengthen outreach and engagement efforts to reduce social isolation for older lesbians in rural communities.

Organizing in rural communities often means the host must provide transportation or initiate carpools to increase access for those who may no longer have the means or ability to drive. In rural areas, with winding unmarked roads, it may mean meeting strangers in a public area to have them follow along in their car. For those seeking a lesbian-specific social event in rural communities, it can require driving two or more hours to attend events. As a result, it may fall upon the host to consider providing overnight accommodations if the weather turns. Strangers can become fast friends when huddling in storm cellars during tornado warnings. Other considerations necessitating overnight accommodations include inebriated guests, festivities running longer than anticipated, or unsafe driving conditions after dark. The more rural the area, the wiser to advise participants to pack an overnight bag just in case and to include any necessary daily medication. The challenge of limited access to resources in other parts of the world becomes a further barrier for attempts in organizing, with many people not having access to transportation or adequate facilities to even host events or gatherings.

In crafting a welcoming space, safety and privacy concerns need to be communicated clearly. Regardless of the gathering, the first question is often about safety. When organizing a backyard BBQ, bonfire and music, lesbian wedding, or game night, often participants would inquire if the neighbors would know it was a "gay" event. Questions about whether rainbow flags would be present or if there will be a privacy fence around the yard reflect a concern for safety. Many rural older lesbians (especially those not out) may also have concerns about who might be in attendance, whether they can trust them not to discuss those in attendance. Some may even check that cars parked at the event don't have bumper stickers that could leave them vulnerable by association. While these concerns may be valid even in urban areas, these fears stem from concern with how individuals might be treated in small rural communities, where sociocultural stigma and repercussions can be harsh if one is dependent on others for assistance, transportation, employment, or housing options. Stigma, driven by homophobia, devalues human beings and contributes to social isolation.[2]

Communication when hosting events should also include discussion about what physical obstacles might impede accessibility. Lesbian festivals and retreats historically endeavored to make events accessible for people with disabilities in ways often neglected in the larger community. For example, Michigan Womyn's Music Festival work crew would nail carpets nap side down over the main trails to create stable pathways and wheelchair access. They would also install handicap accessible showers and portable toilets, provide shuttles between events and campsites, even staff a specific camping site for those requiring assistance. Having someone available to transport luggage and supplies to campsites and sign language interpreters for performances increased accessibility for participants. While not all events can accommodate specific needs, it is helpful for participants to know details so they can make an informed choice in deciding if they are able to attend.

If events are substance-free, this should be clearly communicated, so that participants can plan accordingly. Higher reported rates of alcohol and other drug usage in the lesbian community compared to the general population contributes to health disparities. Older lesbians in recovery may avoid events that revolve around substance use. As environmental toxins increase in our world, chemical sensitives and allergies mean participants appreciate knowing if events will be fragrance-free, or even if pets are allowed.

Claiming a lesbian identity remains a personal struggle for many in rural areas. Identity politics and cultural clashes within the LGBT community often result in heated exchanges over terminology use (womyn-born-womyn, assigned female at birth, raised female, identify female, lesbian, queer, gender nonconforming, butch, femme, dyke, woman who has sex with other women) and whether lesbian spaces are inclusive or exclusive of trans woman. What is often lost in debate over lesbian space is acknowledgment that fear and concerns can be reflective of a woman's lived experiences. For many rural trans women, their pain and struggle for acceptance and affirmation as women drives their need for inclusion, and they may struggle to find open and accepting spaces. Bisexual women, especially those partnered with a man or who are polyamorous, may have concerns about whether they would be welcomed at lesbian events or may anticipate discrimination. For some women, even vocalizing same-sex attraction can be terrifying, especially if they are questioning their identity in later life. Awkward first crushes are difficult to navigate as teenagers, even more so if you've been married to a man for thirty years when you realize you have always been attracted to women. Internalized misogyny can be so deeply ingrained that these women may question the meaning of their lives when coming to terms with a lesbian identity.

A grandmother in her fifties, attending her first ever "lesbian event," shared that she was first married at sixteen, a mother at seventeen, and divorced by twenty-one. She had then married and divorced two other abusive men during her life. She wasn't even sure how to think of herself since, as she said, "How can I be a lesbian if I have never kissed a woman?" She worried her father would no longer speak to her and her adult son would forbid any contact with her grandchild if they ever found out. Another rural lesbian shared she had been raped several times in her life and wanted a space "safe from men, away from penises, without having the air sucked out of a conversation." She suffered from PTSD, waking in cold sweats, even after years of therapy. She sought out lesbian spaces in order to protect herself after a lifetime of having to accommodate men to survive.

Another woman in her seventies shared that, while she was comfortable with her understanding of herself as a lesbian, because of her struggles managing bipolar disorder she was estranged from her family, and her adult child "refused any contact with her." Like many stay-at-home mothers during the 1970s, she had worked temporary positions that rarely offered health insurance or benefit options. Divorced from her husband soon after their marriage and having female partners prior to legal recognition of same-sex marriage, she had limited safety against poverty in her later years with social security. She relocated from a supportive landdyke community in Vermont to Arkansas. Having been single for many years, her health failing, she now felt trapped in a closeted existence in an assisted living facility. Her friends in the area were mainly elderly males in the facility who would drive her to local AA meetings. She knew only a few lesbians in the area, lived in a heavily conservative, religious community, with a limited support network, and only an 812 dollars monthly social security allotment. Like many elders, she had a complicated health history. An emergency room trip for an infected tooth precipitated a financial crisis.

In South Africa, many black families rely heavily on the financial support of working relatives, a concept that is termed "black tax." For older lesbians who were previously married to men and have children from those heterosexual relationships, this financial support is often withheld, as a form of punishment for not conforming to traditional/cultural roles.

For many rural older lesbians, the lifetime effects of the gender pay gap can mean their elder years are defined by poverty, which can exacerbate existing health problems. Accident or illnesses may mean reliance on others for assistance in daily life skills like bathing, cooking, or cleaning. Older lesbians, even those out at other times in their life, may make the difficult choice to cut ties to lesbian culture and community, cancel lesbian magazine subscriptions, give away lesbian music or book collections, destroy photographs or personal mementos, if they become dependent on professional care. This is exacerbated in states and countries without adequate laws to protect older lesbians from discrimination in housing or in health care. Erasure of significant relationships may continue in death. For example, the coauthors of this piece have only seen one joint lesbian gravestone inscribed with "I was her beloved and she was mine."

Housing in rural areas can be limited. Even when housing discrimination laws address sexual orientation or gender identity or expression, landlords may deny older rural lesbians rentals in many countries and U.S. states. Another source of housing stress is the need to find temporary shelter, especially if due to changes in relationship status. Even an amicable breakup can elicit concerns about where to go next, who might be supportive, not just within the lesbian community but among family or community members. Some may simply not have the financial means to live alone. Rural communities may not have emergency housing options for lesbians leaving abusive partners. After a breakup, one woman shared she had "been sleeping in her jeep for a year, since she couldn't afford an apartment on her own." She was estranged from her biological family, who didn't want anything to do with her "lifestyle." She lost her church community and "everything important to her" in coming out. Now, without her ex, her only connection to LGBT community was the yearly Mid-South Pride celebration.

Intimate partner violence occurs in same-sex relationships, but the assumption that an emergency shelter is only needed by women escaping violence perpetrated by male partners has been deeply ingrained in the U.S. domestic violence shelter movement. Some African countries still have outdated patriarchal laws that do not allow women to inherit land. This obviously has significant bearing on women and their livelihood in general but is worse for those who are lesbians.

In the United States, the Violence Against Women Act provides funding for many programs and services. Internationally, the United Nations Handbook for Legislation on Violence Against Women specifically recommends that legislation recognize that women's experience with violence is shaped, in part, by sexual orientation, and that legislation to address violence against women specifically should protect all women, without discrimination based on their sexual orientation.[3]

Rural shelters often neglect consideration of the needs of older lesbian women fleeing violence within their relationships. Issues persist for adequate training and the cultural humility of shelter staff. Practical concerns shared among others experiencing violence may include limited cell phone reception and limited transportation to access shelters. What differs for older rural lesbians are concerns the lesbian community might not believe them, that the lesbian community might support abusive partners, shelter staff assumptions that the person escaping a violent home has a heterosexual partner, threats of being outed to family, employers, or community. Additionally, persistent social and gender expectations for lesbians may contribute to reluctance to end abusive relationships, as well as minimization of the damage and level of violence that can occur within lesbian relationships.

Hate crimes, rapes, and violence specifically targeting older lesbians rarely get reported in rural communities. Disclosure to health care professionals or the police creates the risk of being outed to family, friends, employers, and community members. Misogynistic terrorism of lesbians, incorrectly labeled "corrective rape," is not uncommon throughout our world. In South Africa, with the legacy of apartheid, racial segregation of social services is challenged by high unemployment rates in historically disadvantaged black communities. Stigma and discrimination from health care professionals impact rural black lesbians dependent on a hostile public health care system. While Act 108 of the Constitution of the Republic of South Africa prohibits discrimination based on a person's sexual orientation,[4] negative cultural attitudes demonizing lesbians persist. Those perceived as gender nonconforming, masculine-presenting, or butch lesbians have been targets of violent attacks or even murdered.[5]

After years of responding to lesbians presenting with physical injuries, unwanted pregnancies, or complications from sexually transmitted diseases resulting from brutal attacks and gang rapes in townships near Johannesburg, South Africa, Ntlotleng produced an innovative approach for healing and fostering social support within an isolated lesbian community. She hosted a three-day lesbian retreat, organizing shelter, food, clothes, blankets, links to community resources, and medical care for participants. The retreat included traditional South African healing rituals, music, art and dance, and provided opportunities for the group to discuss the violence they had endured. Especially for butch lesbians, this retreat provided a healing space, affirming identity for those who often endured brutal rapes with little community empathy or means to hold their attackers accountable since they did not conform to gender role expectations, clothing choices, or mannerisms expected for women. This innovative model could easily be implemented in other rural communities around the world for lesbians who experienced similar traumas and lack of social support.

Community building in rural areas requires practical considerations when planning events. Increased social contact in living our lives has helped to change attitudes and social acceptance. Yet rural areas require sensitivity and understanding of the nuances of the risks older lesbians face and support for why they may choose to remain closeted. Individuals can be a catalyst for change within a rural community. Start small and keep it simple. Light candles, set out the food, and enjoy the social connections that board games, BBQs, and music can provide. Potluck dinners, the backbone of lesbian gatherings, help to ease the stress of hosting events. They also allow others to have a means to start a conversation and contribute to cocreation in building community. For many older rural lesbians who cannot rely upon biological families, these communities become family of choice, witnessing life events, attending weddings or funerals. PFLAG groups and affirming religious communities can provide a bridge to support in areas that can be hostile. Linkage to lesbian-specific resources such as *Lesbian Connection*,[6] the *Lesbian Herstory Archives*,[7] and contact information for landdyke communities such as *Maize, a Lesbian Country Magazine*[8] or *Shewolf's Directory of Wimmin's Land and Lesbian Communities*[9] may also help to reduce isolation and provide ongoing social connections to improve the overall health and well-being for older rural lesbians.

It is evident that older rural lesbians face significant sociocultural challenges in the United States and throughout the world, such as limited or poor access to resources, facilities, and, most importantly, support structures. It remains of utmost importance to encourage agency by deeply reflecting on lessons learned and creative strategies already utilized by various women from different settings to create support structures for themselves and their fellow community members. Health care professionals need to support community building efforts, instead of imposing solutions that may not necessarily meet the needs of older rural lesbians. Although many of these women live in stressful circumstances, they continue to live and love, every day, against all odds. This is a true definition of resiliency.

Dr. Kat Carrick is a social worker, activist, and educator based in Pittsburgh, Pennsylvania. She has been involved in both clinical and community social work across the service line, including grassroots activism, community mental health, foster care, inpatient psychiatric care, private practice, hospice care, domestic violence, trauma, and hospital administration. As part of the core faculty for the LGBTQ Health, Policy & Practice Graduate Certificate Program at George Washington University, she developed the Rural Health and Lesbian Health course curriculum, supported program development, and established student scholarships with her grant writing skills. She is an adjunct faculty member for the School of Social Work at Simmons University. She also serves on the Peer Review Committee for the annual conference for GLMA: Health Professionals Advancing LGBT Equality. Her passion is teaching health care professionals how to provide more culturally responsive care to the LGBTQ community. She earned a Doctorate in Social Work and a Doctoral Certificate in Women, Gender, and Sexuality from the University of Pittsburgh, a Master's in Clinical Social Work from Smith College, and a Bachelor's in Psychology from Chatham University.

Dr. Ntlotleng Mabena is public health clinician and an academic based in Johannesburg, South Africa. Her areas of work include HIV management, LGBT health, sexual and reproductive health with special focus on contraceptives and termination of pregnancies, and gender-based violence and rape care. Her LGBT health experience includes clinical management of transgender individuals and advocacy and research relating to women having sex with women's HIV risks, rape, and mental health needs, among others. Dr. Mabena also works with Clinical Forensic Medicine department in the Johannesburg District, providing medical care to survivors of sexual violence and domestic violence, providing training to both clinical and law enforcement staff on the comprehensive management of assault cases, and as an expert witnesses in court. Dr. Mabena is currently working on her organization called Open House Initiative, to implement responses to some identified health needs and systems improvement through collaboration with relevant stakeholders to ensure care and guarantee that justice is served.

Notes

1. Parents and Friends of Lesbians and Gays (PFLAG) is a national nonprofit organization in the United States, with local chapters throughout the U.S.
2. Stephen E. Gilman, Susan D. Cochran, Vickie M. Mays, Michael Hughes, David Ostrow, and Ronald C. Kessler, "Risk of Psychiatric Disorders among Individuals Reporting Same-Sex Sexual Partners in the National Comorbidity Survey," *American Journal of Public Health* 91, no. 6 (June 2001): 933–39, accessed June 5, 2019, https://www.ncbi.nlm.nih.gov/pmc/articles/PMC1446471/pdf/11392937.pdf.
3. United Nations Department of Economic and Social Affairs, Division for the Advancement of Women, Handbook for Legislation on Violence against Women (New York: United Nations, 2009).
4. Constitution of the Republic of South Africa no. 108 of 1996, accessed June 5, 2019, https://www.gov.za/sites/default/files/images/a108-96.pdf.
5. Zethu Matebeni, "Exploring Black Lesbian Sexualities and Identities in Johannesburg" (PhD diss., University of Witwatersrand, Johannesburg), accessed June 5, 2019, http://wiredspace.wits.ac.za/bitstream/handle/10539/10274/Matebeni%20PhD%20thesis%202011.pdf?sequence=2.
6. Lesbian Connection, accessed June 5, 2019, http://www.lconline.org.
7. Lesbian Herstory Archives, accessed June 5, 2019, http://www.lesbianherstoryarchives.org/.
8. *Maize, a Lesbian Country Magazine*, see Women, Earth & Spirit, Inc., accessed June 5, 2019, http://womanearthandspirit.org/.
9. *Shewolf's Directory of Wimmin's Lands and Lesbian Communities (2013–2016)*, 6th edition, email shewolforiginal@aol.com, see Lesbian Natural Resources, accessed June 5, 2019, http://www.lesbiannaturalresources.org/publications/.

21

Caregiving Concerns for LGBT Older Adults

Liz Bradbury

When a professional specializing in older adult care says, "Of course we are LGBT-supportive, we treat *everyone* the same!" it's a big red flag.

Simply put, older LGBT adults are *not* the same as everyone else. Even when an institution or individual is not intending to be exclusive, saying "we treat everyone equally" indicates that the older LGBT adult client or patient's needs will probably not be met.

I am an older LGBT adult myself. I can say with certainty our life experiences and needs are different from older adults who are not LGBT. They're also different from LGBT adults who are younger. Lack of knowledge about older LGBT adult lives and culture can cause providers to create barriers to care. This occurs, often unintentionally, by simply using the wrong words, saying the wrong things, lacking inclusive policies, not using current best practices, or just not listening.

The remedy is simple: learn about the unique needs that older LGBT adults have and be prepared to apply that knowledge when working with this population.

The older LGBT adult population is rapidly growing, but protocols often ignore the factors that make older LGBT adults more likely to need institutional care and less likely to be able to age in place.

Due to the baby boomer population bubble, every day another ten thousand people in the U.S. turn sixty-five.[1] About 55 million Americans are age sixty-five or older, and, by 2050, an estimated 86.7 million will be over sixty-five.[2] That's a 38 percent increase.

Within that growing population there are about 2.8 million older LGBT adults over sixty-five.[3] By 2030, that number will double.[4] Yet while the percentage of aging LGBT people within the baby boomer population is already a large demographic, there is more to consider when estimating the need for health care professionals trained to work with the aging LGBT population.

Most older people would prefer to age in their own homes as long as possible.[5] In fact, 87 percent of adults age sixty-five or older want to stay in their current home and community as they age.[6] It's easy to conclude that an older LGBT adult might feel more in control in their own home and less likely to find their identity challenged. Further, "aging in place" is not only better for an older person's general sense of wellness, it's often less expensive than institutional care.[7]

Older adults need help from others in order to age in place. Everything from installing the window air conditioner unit to help with dressing and bathing are needs that can be met at home by "informal care." Informal care is generally defined as the unpaid care provided to older and dependent people by a person with whom they have a social relationship, such as a spouse, parent, child, other relative, neighbor, friend, or other nonrelative.[8]

In the United States, 96 percent of all informal care is provided by adult children, spouses, grandchildren, the spouses of adult children, and other relatives.[9] The American Association of Retired Persons (AARP) acknowledges this in its mainstream booklet, *Prepare to Care—A Planning Guide for Families.*[10] Of the ten photo illustrations in this helpful booklet, eight show an older adult with a caregiver who is their daughter, one picture shows a caregiver son, and one shows both a son and daughter (in-law). The adult children caregivers look the same as the parents; they are the same race and even have the same hair color.

Agencies advocating for older adults assert that any older person could become an "elder orphan." An elder orphan is someone who is aging alone with no family available to help them with their everyday caregiving needs. Research indicates that anyone might become an elder orphan, but specific circumstances increase the risk. See those risk factors, as they compare between older LGBT adults and the majority population:

Who is at risk for becoming an elder orphan?[11]

- Single older adults with no or limited social circles and support groups.
- Older women without support.

- Older adults estranged from siblings and family.
- Single older adults with no children.
- Single older adults with estranged children.
- Childless couples.
- Married couples with estranged children.
- Older adults who are isolated.

LGBT older adults are[12]

- Twice as likely to age as a single person.
- Twice as likely to reside alone.
- More likely to be estranged from (some or all) family.
- Four times less likely to have children.
- More likely to be isolated.

Though many LGBT people do have children, spouses, and birth families, older LGBT adults' statistical risk factors of becoming elder orphans are more significant than those of the general public. Consider that older LGBT adults are four times less likely to have children, are far more likely to have been ostracized by family, and are twice as likely to live alone, and you begin to understand the potential disparity of informal care options.

Mainstream folks are always quick to point out that just because you have kids doesn't mean they are going to take care of you. Yet 96 percent of all informal care in the U.S. is provided by relatives, and about 34.2 million Americans have provided unpaid care to an adult over fifty in the last twelve months.[13] So it's obvious that many adult children are providing care for their aging parents. *Only 4 percent of these caregivers are not relatives or family.* Recently I attended a presentation on The Conversation Project—a project dedicated to helping older people express their wishes for end-of-life care. The presenter spoke eloquently to the large audience on talking with your adult children about end-of-life issues. In every sentence she described how to broach this sensitive subject with your daughters and sons. The group of older lesbians I was sitting with began to fold their arms and shake their heads.

Finally, someone from another part of the auditorium asked, "But what if you don't have any family?" The presenter responded, "Well, then have this conversation with your friends or your nieces and nephews." Apparently, she didn't grasp the concept that nieces and nephews were actually family. In the next breath, the presenter returned to talking about adult children and didn't get off that track for the rest of the evening. It made me and the other childless attendees feel as though this project had nothing to do with us.

I was asked to join a government-led community group working on aging issues in my two-county area. In a large meeting, I suggested that we stop using language that implied all older people would be cared for by their children. I explained that I was representing the LGBT community in this group, and we are far less likely to have children to care for us as we age. The facilitator simply skipped over my comment and ignored my suggestion. The adult children model of care is so ingrained into senior care protocol, that many care professionals cannot think of it in any other way. The remedy is simple: end the presumption that adult children or family will be available to care for older LGBT adults and plan accordingly.

•

LGBT people are more likely to be informal caregivers. Among all informal caregivers, 9 percent self-identify as LGBT.[14] That 9 percent is more than double the estimated percentage of LGBT people in the general population.[15]

LGBT-identified male caregivers report providing more hours of care than female caregivers. The average weekly hours of care provided by females from both the LGBT and general population is similar (twenty-six vs. twenty-eight hours), but LGBT males provide far more hours of care than males who do not identify as LGBT (forty-one vs. twenty-nine hours). Further, 14 percent of gay males indicate that they are full-time caregivers, spending over 150 hours per week in this capacity, compared to 3 percent of lesbian and 2 percent of woman-identified bisexual survey respondents.[16]

More simply put, daughters, whether they are heterosexual and cisgender or LGBT, are more than twice as likely to take care of their aging parents than heterosexual sons. But LGBT-identified sons are about eight times more likely than heterosexual sons to be caregivers.[17] (Takeaway: if you want to be sure to be taken care of in your old age either have a lot of daughters or a few gay sons.)

While the mainstream AARP caregiver guide shows many photos of daughters, it only shows one picture of a son caring for a parent. Based on these caregiver statistics the likelihood that this caregiver is a gay son is eight to one. While senior care facilities should include positive programs and policies with LGBT residents and patients in mind, it's just as important to recognize that caregivers, especially male caregivers, are very likely to be LGBT, and will expect facilities to be LGBT-friendly and culturally competent. The remedy is simple: understand that there is a high percentage of LGBT people who are informal and family caregivers. Senior care agencies should professionally train all administrators and staff to be culturally competent on LGBT issues.

A recent survey found that three out of four LGBT adults age forty-five and older say they are concerned about having enough support from family and friends as they age.[18] Because older LGBT adults are less likely to have family support, nearly all health and welfare literature that addresses LGBT aging issues indicates that older LGBT adults often rely on "families of choice" for their informal and supportive care.

Prepare to Care: A Planning Guide for Caregivers in the LGBT Community, a booklet specifically for the LGBT population, defines these caregivers as "diverse family structures that include but are not limited to life partners, close friends, and other loved ones who are not biologically related or legally recognized but who provide social and caregiving support to an individual."[19] This informative planning guide created by AARP with SAGE, the national organization advocating for LGBT older adults, presents valuable information, and what it says about families of choice is absolutely correct. Agencies and organizations all over the world that present information on the needs of older LGBT adults frequently state that a family of choice is a possible caregiving solution for many older LGBT adults.

However, the families of choice model is extremely problematic as the presumptive default caregiving solution! Consider that LGBT people of the baby boomer generation have life experiences that include:

- Denial of legal and societal recognition of our relationships.
- Tremendous barriers when seeking to have or adopt children.
- Denial of health care in the face of a terrible epidemic.
- Ridicule by religious institutions of our relationships.
- Not just estrangement from but ostracization by our families.
- Being treated as outsiders by society.
- Employment discrimination and housing loss when we were honest about our relationships.

Understand that for most of the lives of older LGBT adults, mainstream society did everything it could to isolate LGBT people and keep us from forming lasting relationships, yet today nearly every protocol for our care in our senior years suggests we *go out and create our own family*. And to top off this irony, nearly every protocol presumes we have already done that!

Having families of choice as caregivers is a great idea. And some older LGBT adults can achieve it. In fact, during the AIDS epidemic in the 1980s, those who were sick and dying were often shunned by their birth families, and loving families of choice emerged to provide care. Those 1980s families of choice are the same LGBT generation that are becoming the older adults of today. But here's the problem: families of choice are made up of friends. In the 1980s, we baby boomers were in our thirties—and so were our friends. When one is eighty, those same friends are around eighty too. They often can't provide the kind of informal care another older person needs. Informal care requires devoted younger people. To have a set of caring friends who are twenty or more years younger is very hard to maintain, let alone create. Presuming that all LGBT people have a family of choice puts older LGBT adults at risk.

Just as the AARP mainstream *Prepare to Care* booklet shows photos that indicate that it's adult daughters who are likely to be their parents' caregivers, *Prepare to Care: A Planning Guide for Caregivers in the LGBT Community* tells its own story in pictures. It acknowledges in its photos that creating a family of choice when one is older is a very hard thing to do. Nearly all the photos of the older LGBT people in this guide show the caregiver as their partner or spouse. While many LGBT people do end up as caregivers for their partner or spouse, there's an inherent problem. An older adult partner or spouse, if one has one, is rarely a generation younger, and is therefore less able to provide informal care.

That means that unless programs successfully help older LGBT adults create and maintain families of choice, they will more likely have to pay for skilled care or will have to enter skilled care facilities at a younger age. There are two remedies for this: first, we must end the presumption that older LGBT adults have families of choice to care for them as they age; and, second, we must create programs that expressly aim to build families of choice for older LGBT adults.

•

Unfortunately, some health care professionals do not believe they need to receive professional training on older LGBT adult health and cultural issues. Lack of awareness and training frequently creates barriers to care and minority stress. In some instances, lack of training or not following best practice protocols seriously harms older LGBT adults. A large 2018 survey found:

- 88 percent of older LGBT adults say they would feel more comfortable with providers who are specifically trained in LGBT patient needs.
- 86 percent want providers to use advertising to highlight LGBT-friendly services.
- 85 percent would prefer to have some staff members who are LGBT themselves.
- 82 percent want providers to display LGBT-welcoming signs or symbols in facilities and online.[20]

During a recent panel I facilitated for doctors, nurses, and other professionals at a major hospital network, an older transgender adult patient recounted the stress she felt when hospital staff refused to use her chosen name and appropriate pronouns and refused to acknowledge her gender. This happened even though she had clearly explained her gender identity, name, and pronouns to her physician and the staff on several occasions, and her gender identity information was in her chart. When she expressed her concern in a phone call, she explained that as a patient she felt that the constant and unapologetic disregard for her gender identity verged on discrimination. She suggested the staff receive some kind of training. A few minutes later, she received an angry return call from the physician himself, insisting that she explain exactly what this discrimination had been. Before the patient could even finish a sentence, the physician cut her off. He sternly told her at length that she was wrong, and that she could no longer be his patient.

When an older transgender adult's transition is not supported it puts their mental and physical health at risk. A Canadian and U.S. study shows access to transition-related health care lowers the risk of suicide by nearly 80 percent. Yet many health care professionals are not only unfamiliar with transgender health issues, but also are not LGBT culturally competent.[21]

Furthermore, 34 percent of all older LGBT adults reported being at least somewhat worried about having to hide their LGBT identity in order to have access to suitable housing options as they age, and among transgender and gender expansive participants, that statistic increases to 54 percent.[22]

These worries develop from a fear that the people in charge of their care as they age may be anti-LGBT. Older LGBT adults have lived through decades of severe discrimination. In their lifetimes they could have been put in jail or mental institutions for being gay. Transgender people are still frequently victims of violence and murder simply because of their gender identity.

Fear that those providing care may fundamentally believe LGBT people are immoral, commit child abuse, or are likely to sexually assault others may cause this population to hide their identities. Those who are HIV positive fear discrimination, stigma, and lack of education. *And these fears are not unfounded.*

In 2019, an older lesbian couple who had been together for fifty years and legally married for ten was denied housing in a senior living community because their relationship violated its cohabitation policy that defined marriage as, "the union of one man and one woman, as marriage is understood in the Bible."[23]

While LGBT people may be able to find supportive older adult care, having to search for a welcoming facility is a factor of minority stress. Heterosexual couples don't have to ask at every care facility if their gender will cause staff to judge their fifty-year relationships as an abomination. There is a simple remedy for this: agencies providing older adult care should adopt LGBT-inclusive policies and programs and professionally train their administrators and staff on cultural competency for the LGBT older adult population.

There are also unique circumstances that affect older LGBT adults.

Legal Marriage

Older LGBT adults who are in long-term committed relationships have many positive reasons to legally marry. In most U.S. states, when one member of a long-term committed couple dies the survivor is at risk for enormous and possibly devastating inheritance tax bills if the couple was not legally married. One eighty-two-year-old gay man I spoke with received a tax bill of 140 thousand dollars, because his uninformed lawyer didn't advise him to simply marry his partner of fifty years, before he died.

Couples get survivor inheritance tax benefits, survivor pensions, social security, burial and decision-making, more than 1,100 statutory federal rights and hundreds of state rights that come with legal marriage. Unless one of the partners would lose disability insurance or a pension from a previous partner, unless they have very high incomes or disparate incomes that could result in higher taxes, or unless they are profoundly against marriage and can afford the financial burden lack of marriage will cause, there are very few reasons for older same-sex couples in long-term committed relationships not to marry.

Consider Robert, who spoke in a recent older LGBT adult health care consumer panel I moderated. Robert lost his beloved partner of twenty-five years, Steve, to cancer. He recounted that on more than one occasion, a doctor or other professional would turn to him in Steve's hospital room and ask rudely, "Who are you?" Robert's response was, "I'm his husband." Which immediately established his legal right to be there.

Robert says the experience of losing his cherished husband was profoundly hard, but he also said that he could not imagine what it would have been like had he and Steve not been legally married. Without legal marriage the government sees people in long-term relationships as "strangers." Even with proxies, wills, and legal powers of attorney, an unmarried partner has very few rights. And no rights at all to make a burial decision after the partner's death. Don't think marriage between older LGBT adults is just something cute—it's essential for health and well-being.

Alzheimer's Disease and Dementia

A recent study on Alzheimer's disease has produced surprising preliminary data showing that while the mainstream population experiences Alzheimer's and other dementias at about 10 percent of the population, dementia affects about 7.4 percent of the LGBT population over sixty-five. Though the raw data does not suggest a disparity for the LGBT community in *risk* for dementia, clear disparities exist due to the lack of culturally appropriate care. In general, the information in this chapter applies to any older LGBT adult whether they have dementia or not. Consider that for long-term same-sex couples, if one partner has dementia, the ability for the committed partner to provide and make judgments about care may become impossible for the caregiver if the couple is not legally married.

As an older LGBT adult myself, with a history of Alzheimer's in my family, including my mother having early onset, my biggest fear is the inability to make decisions for myself. I can confidently say that for me, awareness and the quality of my life is far more important than longevity.

Transgender Veterans

Statistics show that transgender people are twice as likely to be veterans than the mainstream population. Among transgender women over sixty-five, one in two are veterans. As a result, many older transgender adults are getting their health care from Veteran's Affairs (VA). It is critical that VA hospitals provide culturally responsive and inclusive care for LGBT older adults, and that health care professionals who work for the VA are trained specifically on the unique health needs of transgender older adults.

Older LGBT adult veterans have endured decades of institutional discrimination. "Don't Ask, Don't Tell" put LGBT people in the armed forces at risk every day. Continued government efforts to attack the rights of transgender service members create profound minority stress. My sister-in-law was a Korean War era career marine and a lesbian. Into her eighties she feared the government would revoke her pension if she was out, decades after her honorable discharge. LGBT veterans need to know they are safe to be honest about their lives to their health care professionals, especially when they receive care at the VA.

In conclusion, the caregiving challenges for older LGBT adults are significant. LGBT older adults are seeking and require care professionals who have the skills, policies, and resources to meet unique LGBT needs. Health care institutions and professionals who welcome LGBT older adults but are not committed to professional LGBT cultural competency training may spark barriers to care. High quality patient-centered care requires cultural and linguistic training. Without specific LGBT training, "LGBT-welcoming" is a hollow description.

Liz Bradbury is the director of the Training Institute at Bradbury-Sullivan LGBT Community Center, where she has presented hundreds of trainings on LGBT issues tailored to the needs of widely diverse groups and organizations. Over her forty-year career as an LGBT activist and advocate she has helped to craft and pass LGBT civil rights legislation in ten municipalities in Pennsylvania, has been called on as an expert on LGBT issues by government agencies and radio and television, has written inclusive policies for major corporations, has been an executive director and leader to several successful, long running LGBT community organizations, published an LGBT newspaper for nineteen years, and has run an LGBT infoline for twenty-five years. She served for fifteen years on the Allentown Human Relations Commission (including three years as chair), where she wrote the guidelines for discrimination investigations and trained investigators. She has authored over four hundred published articles and columns on LGBT issues. She and her spouse and partner of thirty-two years, Patricia Sullivan, live in Allentown, Pennsylvania.

Notes

1 Russell Heimlich, "Baby Boomers Retire," Pew Research Center, December 29, 2010, accessed June 5, 2019, http://www.pewresearch.org/fact-tank/2010/12/29/baby-boomers-retire/.

2 Jennifer M. Ortman, Victoria A. Velkoff, and Howard Hogan, "An Aging Nation: The Older Population in the United States," *Current Population Reports* (May 2014), accessed June 5, 2019, https://www.census.gov/prod/2014pubs/p25-1140.pdf.

3 "Lesbian, Gay, Bisexual and Transgender Aging," American Psychological Association, accessed June 5, 2019, https://www.apa.org/pi/lgbt/resources/aging.

4 "Sixty-Five Plus in the United States." U.S. Census Bureau, May 1995, accessed June 5, 2019, https://www.census.gov/population/socdemo/statbriefs/agebrief.html.

5 "Making Home Safe and Accessible for Seniors," American Psychological Association, 2002, unavailable June 5, 2019, doi:10.1037/e439292008-002.

6 Cheryl Lampkin, "What is Livable? Community Preferences of Older Adults," *AARP Public Policy Institute*, April 2014, accessed June 5, 2019, https://www.aarp.org/content/dam/aarp/research/public_policy_institute/liv_com/2014/what-is-livable-ib-AARP-ppi-liv-com.pdf.

7 "5 Benefits of Aging in Place," Retirement Living, May 10, 2019, accessed June 5, 2019, https://www.retirementliving.com/5-benefits-of-aging-in-place.

8 Judy Triantafillou et al., "Informal Care in the Long-Term Care System," *Interlinks*, September 2011, accessed June 5, 2019, http://interlinks.euro.centre.org/sites/default/files/WP5%20Informal%20care_ExecutiveSummary_FINAL_1.pdf.

9 Marc A. Cohen, Maurice Weinrobe, and Jessica Miller, "Informal Caregivers of Disabled Elders with Long-Term Care Insurance," *ASPE*, January 2000, accessed June 5, 2019, https://aspe.hhs.gov/basic-report/informal-caregivers-disabled-elders-long-term-care-insurance.

10 AARP, *Prepare to Care—A Planning Guide for Families*, accessed June 5, 2019, https://www.aarp.org/content/dam/aarp/home-and-family/caregiving/2012-10/PrepareToCare-Guide-FINAL.pdf.

11 "Living without Family: 5 Stages of Self Care Seniors Should Know," SeniorLiving.org, accessed June 5, 2019, https://www.seniorliving.org/health/aging/no-family/.

12 "Caregiver Statistics: Demographics," *Family Caregiver Alliance*, April 17, 2019, accessed June 5, 2019, https://www.caregiver.org/caregiver-statistics-demographics.

13 Ibid.

14 Ibid.

15 Frank Newport, "In U.S., Estimate of LGBT Population Rises to 4.5%," Gallup, May 22, 2018, accessed June 5, 2019, https://news.gallup.com/poll/234863/estimate-lgbt-population-rises.aspx.

16 "Caregiver Statistics: Demographics."

17 Ibid.

18 Angela Houghton, "Maintaining Dignity: A Survey of LGBT Adults Age 45 and Older," AARP, March 2018, accessed June 5, 2019, https://www.aarp.org/research/topics/life/info-2018/maintaining-dignity-lgbt.html.

19 SAGE/AARP, *Prepare to Care: A Planning Guide for Caregivers in the LGBT Community*, accessed June 5, 2019, https://www.aarp.org/content/dam/aarp/home-and-family/caregiving/2017/05/prepare-to-care-guide-lgbt-aarp.pdf.

20 Houghton, "Maintaining Dignity."

21 Greta R. Bauer, Ayden I. Bauer, Jake Pyne, Robb Travers, and Rebecca Hammond, "Intervenable Factors Associated with Suicide Risk in Transgender Persons: A Respondent Driven Sampling Study in Ontario, Canada," *BMC Public Health* 15, no. 525 (June 2015), accessed June 5, 2019, https://bmcpublichealth.biomedcentral.com/articles/10.1186/s12889-015-1867-2.

22 Houghton, "Maintaining Dignity."

23 Nick Duffy, "Elderly Lesbian Couple Rejected from Retirement Community Because They Are Married," PinkNews, July 26, 2018, accessed June 5, 2019, https://www.pinknews.co.uk/2018/07/26/elderly-lesbian-couple-retirement-community/.

22

Housing and Health for LGBT Older Adults

Imani Woody

I'm pretty sure when U.S. actress Bette Davis said, "Getting old ain't for sissies," she was not referring to gay older adults specifically but to the challenges that aging can bring to us all, no matter our sexual orientation or gender identity. *Old* is not the destination to be traveling in our youth-obsessed culture. The politics of age have made growing old with maladies almost feel like a crime, something we are not ready to "cop" to—therefore making many of us invisible.

I remember when my then seventy-eight-year-old stepmother asked me who I was calling old, when I referred to her and some of her peers as old! Getting there myself, old age can be particularly challenging for LGBT same-gender loving (SGL) baby boomers and older adults born during the Silent Generation.[1]

As a matter of fact, baby boomers began turning sixty-five in 2011 and are now driving growth at the older ages of the population. By 2029, when all the baby boomers will be sixty-five years and over, more than 20 percent of the total U.S. population will be over the age of sixty-five. The American Psychological Association states that more than 39 million people in the U.S. are age sixty-five years or older, including 2.4 million people who identify as LGBT.

We all have heard that fifty is the new forty . . . and Disrupt Aging. As if living to be fifty years old and getting older are not only biological markers of the human species but gifts. Ageism is hardwired into our institutional systems and can systematically attack from inside (internal ageism) and outside. Ageism is insidious and can be mean-spirited. It can cripple one's self-esteem and limit access to housing, social services, and societal integration. If you have lived to be in your fifth decade, you have probably experienced ageism. If you are an older woman, you probably began to experience it in your forties. If you are an older gay male, ageism may have knocked on your door in your thirties. Ageism, like racism, sexism, and heterosexism, systematically regulates people toward "the back of the bus." In 1969, Robert N. Butler, MD, a former chair of the DC Advisory Committee on Aging, coined the word "ageism." He noted that "ageism can be seen as a systematic stereotyping of and discrimination against people because they are old, just as racism and sexism accomplish this with skin color and gender."[2] Ageism is so prevalent that many older LGBT/SGL folks are going back into the closet, because being gay and being old is just too hard.

One sixty-seven-year-old African American lesbian elder cited her experience: "Well, I would say that getting older in this country is difficult because we have no reverence for the elderly, which is not true in a lot of cultures. So when you add another . . . stigma to it now, not only am I old, I'm old, I'm an old African-American female. And females in this country, at least my experience has been that you don't enjoy the same reverence as males do and then when you add African American to that, then it's even less. So now, I'm already down pretty far, and then when you add being a lesbian to that, that puts you in the toilet."[3]

The experiences of an LGBT elder born in the Silent Generation of McCarthyism can be quite different from the experiences of a LGBT baby boomer reared in the times of the Stonewall riots and the Civil Rights Movements. However, both generations of LGBT/SGL elders have experienced injurious events and rejection that have caused many to conceal their sexual orientation and gender identity.[4] In the final analysis, these factors have had an adverse effect on much of this cohort's ability to access social and community-based services, often creating unwarranted barriers and increased health concerns. Recent research has shown that LGBT/SGL people are more likely to experience depression, increased isolation, and loneliness because of the stigma, prejudice, and discrimination related to aging in a youth-oriented society.[5]

Here is the voice of a sixty-year-old Black transgender woman: "I'm the biggest advocate for my own care, but frequently it can be frustrating, extremely frustrating. . . . I had an incident with one of the case managers at a large medical facility and when I tried to report it, it seemed like no one wanted to hear it. I completely lost medical coverage and benefits from 2010 to 2011 and it was really frustrating to get it back. For about four months I had nothing and tried to explain that my health was in jeopardy. I need medicine for my heart, and I have diabetes. I contacted the Center for Medicare Services, but they weren't always helpful. . . . I just want to be as healthy as I can be and sometimes, I get tired, mentally, emotionally, and physically. If I were younger, I don't think I would be dismissed so easily. You can see the look on their face when they just think you're being cranky and old."

The gross discrimination and stigma can produce such fear that many LGBT/SGL elders are invisible. Many elders in my research cited "a need to know stance" when deciding to share their sexual orientation or gender identity with professionals and family. Many waited until they were in their forties or fifties before sharing this important information with their families. Many did not share with their medical team because of the perceived stigma associated with coming out, especially among gay men. A sixty-three-year-old gay man stated, "You have to be careful because the minute you tell a medical person you are gay, they automatically in 90% of the cases will assume you are HIV positive and start to react that way. And I have had to remind a doctor or two, I'm not positive, I'm negative. I'm gay but I'm negative. So let's stop that train of thought right now!"

Studies comparing key health indicators based on sexual orientation found that LGBT midlife and older adults experience disparities in regard to disability, cardiovascular disease, obesity, stress, and physical health.[6] Other studies show that transgender older adults experience the highest rates of victimization; the highest death rate because of victimization is experienced by transgender women of color. Emotional distress and social isolation are two of the largest threats to health for LGBT/SGL elders and are exacerbated by perceptions of having been treated badly or discriminated against or perceptions that they were going to be treated badly or discriminated against because others thought they were LGBT/SGL. There has been empirical evidence of medical professionals not wanting to provide services to LGBT/SGL people.

LGBT/SGL people are the largest subcategory of all demographics, because they are members of all groups. They include African American, Latinx, Asian, Caucasian, Middle Eastern, Christian, Muslim, Buddhist, young people, old people, people with dementia, caregivers, moms, grandparents, actors, doctors, retirees, lawyers, pastors, and senators. However, many mainstream health and provider service organizations, wellness centers, and retirement communities routinely state that they do not have any LGBT/SGL people on their census or as clients. When an agency states they don't have LGBT/SGL older adults, they set up a culture of invisibility that can also grow into a culture of oppression for clients and staff alike. Not seeing oneself reflected in the business of the organization can leave LGBT/SGL older adults vulnerable when they are the population most in need of these services to ensure a quality life in old age.

A lifetime of discrimination has reduced the support networks and economic security of many of our LGBT/SGL elders, leaving them vulnerable to housing instability at a critical point in their lives, and many are priced out of housing. The federal guideline states that when 30 percent of your income is for housing, it is a "housing burden"; while paying 50 percent of your income for housing is considered a "severe burden." In many states, a one-bedroom apartment costs more than 100 percent of a social security check.[7]

Research and experience show that when LGBT/SGL people apply for housing in independent senior living communities or attempt to rent and buy apartments and homes, they routinely encounter discrimination, and their housing choices become even starker. A recent national investigation confirmed that almost half (48 percent) of older same-sex couples experienced at least one form of adverse differential treatment when inquiring about housing; one in four transgender older Americans report discrimination when seeking housing; and 78 percent of older LGBT people are interested in LGBT-friendly affordable housing.[8]

Mary's House for Older Adults was created to address this lack of housing. We believe that the lack of affordable housing is a public health issue. We believe that without stable housing, elders are unable to focus on any other issues. We know the problem of unaffordability is increasing. We at Mary's House routinely receive cries for help for housing for an LGBT/SGL elder who is approaching eviction, who can no longer "couch surf" with his friend, whose housing has been sold to developers.

Recently a case manager wrote, "I recently learned about Mary's House for Older Adults through an Internet search. I am currently working with a 60 year-old man who is gay, homeless, and an undocumented immigrant. He is in need of housing and supportive social services and his options are limited by his immigration status. Can you help?"

And a seventy-something lesbian who has led an amazing life contacted us. (She was standing a couple of rows from Rev. Dr. Martin Luther King when he gave his "I Have a Dream" speech). Her current residence is being sold by the owner. She can't do a huge number of stairs and can afford about 400 to 450 dollars per month. She was asking, "Can you help?"

And we try. We provide information and referrals and coordinate access to government and local programs. However, we also know that there will never be enough affordable, culturally competent housing to support the grey tsunami of LGBT/SGL elders. We know that the education of the existing residences and providers for culturally competent care is paramount to eliminating barriers to care. Our first residence is a model of communal living and will be a fifteen single-room occupancy residence in Washington, DC. This model will be replicated on smaller scales throughout the United States. We are eliminating barriers and creating families—one house at a time.

Housing is a social determinant of health, and housing is a human right.

Dr. Imani Woody is the founding director and CEO of Mary's House for Older Adults, Inc. She has a PhD in Human Services, specializing in nonprofit management. Her thesis is titled *Lift Every Voice: A Qualitative Exploration of Ageism and Heterosexism as Experienced by Older African American Lesbian Women and Gay Males When Addressing Social Services Needs.* She holds an MA in Human Services from Lincoln University and is a graduate of Georgetown University's paralegal program. Dr. Woody has been an advocate of women, people of color, and LGBT/SGL issues for more than twenty years and is a member of the National LGBT Elder Housing Initiative and the DC Mayors World Health Organization Age-Friendly Cities Commission. She is also the program officer for the Older Adults Advisory Council for Metropolitan Community Churches and a board member of the LGBT Technology Partnership. She lives with her wife of seventeen years in Brookland, Washington, DC.

Notes

1 Same-gender loving is an identity claimed by some African Americans to describe gay or bisexual behavior; the baby boomer generation is defined as those born between 1946 and 1964; the Silent Generation is defined as those born between 1925 and 1945.

2 W. Andrew Achenbaum, "A History of Ageism Since 1969," American Society on Aging, accessed June 6, 2019, https://www.asaging.org/blog/history-ageism-1969.

3 Imani Woody, "Aging Out: Exploring Ageism and Heterosexism among African American Lesbians and Gay Males," American Society on Aging, accessed June 6, 2019, https://www.asaging.org/blog/aging-out-exploring-ageism-and-heterosexism-among-african-american-lesbians-and-gay-males.

4 Robert M. Kertzner, Ilan H. Meyer, David M. Frost, and Michael J. Stirratt, "Social and Psychological Well-Being in Lesbians, Gay Men, and Bisexuals: The Effects of Race, Gender, Age, and Sexual Identity," *American Journal of Orthopsychiatry* 79, no. 4 (October 2009): 500–10, accessed June 2, 2019, https://www.ncbi.nlm.nih.gov/pubmed/20099941.

5 Imani Woody, "Aging Out: A Qualitative Exploration of Ageism and Heterosexism among Aging African American Lesbians and Gay Men," *Journal of Homosexuality* 61, no. 1 (January 2014): 145–65.

6 Karen I. Fredrikesen-Goldsen, Hyun-Jun Kim, Susan E. Barkan, Anna Muraco, and Charles P. Hoy-Ellis, "Health Disparities among Lesbian, Gay Male and Bisexual Older Adults: Results from a Population-Based Study," *American Journal of Public Health* 103, no. 10 (October 2013): 1802–9, accessed June 6, 2019, https://www.ncbi.nlm.nih.gov/pmc/articles/PMC3770805/.

7 SAMHSA, "Transcript: Housing Instability Risk: How to Recognize It and What to Do When You See It," accessed June 6, 2019, https://www.samhsa.gov/sites/default/files/programs_campaigns/recovery_to_practice/transcript-homelessness_1_20171004.pdf.

8 *Opening Doors: An Investigation of Barriers to Senior Housing for Same-Sex Couples* (Washington, DC: Equal Rights Center, 2014), accessed June 6, 2019, https://equalrightscenter.org/wp-content/uploads/senior_housing_report.pdf.

23

Grieving Together: LGBT Bereavement Support Groups

Justin Sabia-Tanis

During my intake interview, I asked how the other members of a grief support group at our local hospice might respond to having a gay man in the mix. The facilitator replied, "Don't worry . . . by the second week, no one will even think twice about your being different. Grief is a great equalizer." And it turned out to be true. For eight weeks, I was the one man, the only queer, in a roomful of straight women as we processed our grief. For most of us, our significant others had died; a couple had lost a beloved parent. Grief was, in fact, a great equalizer. After a little—fairly well-disguised—surprise at my presence on the first night, we bonded, as you are supposed to, and focused on the difficult, rewarding, bewildering, painful journey of grieving together.

My experiences and insights were part of the group dynamics and people went out of their way to ensure that I was truly included. I genuinely felt that the group members did not, in fact, see me as particularly different. I was the same as everyone else. Here lies the crux of the problem—my differences and those of queer culture were neither seen nor even acknowledged as existing. I felt that to insist on giving them space would have broken the social contract by which we were sharing our common experiences of grieving. At the same time, when LGBT experiences of grieving are often minimized because our relationships are still sometimes considered less important or less meaningful, the experience of being respected as an equal griever was a positive validation of my loss. I was the same as everyone else.

In this chapter, I will briefly describe my own experiences of grief as an LGBT person, along with some reflections from my work as a pastoral caregiver and academic working in the field of LGBT and queer studies. In particular, I will note what some of the unique features of grieving are among LGBT people and what might help foster healthy and healing responses to significant loss.

I am a gay transgender man whose non-transgender, pansexual, polyamorous partner died in 2009 following open heart surgery. His last days were spent in a hospital in central Virginia. In the intensive care unit, as he was dying, visitation was limited to "family," which did not legally include me or other members of his chosen family. Fortunately, his son was very supportive of my presence, and the staff looked the other way, but there was the constant fear that I would be blocked from visiting him. Both this process and his death were traumatic for me; they were shattering, in fact.

Grieving itself is a strange experience of dislocation. It is, of course, a normal process, part of almost every human life. Everything that lives will eventually die and end its physical existence on this earth. All of the people, animals, and plants that we love will die and leave us if we don't leave them first. Grieving should be a common human experience. But, of course, in modern Western culture, it often is seen as an aberration, a reminder of emotional pain, and socially uncomfortable. I was recently approached by a first-year college student in one of my classes who was bewildered by the fact that he was having trouble focusing on his school work since his grandmother had died; the two had been close. When I asked how long he had been having difficulty, he told me that she had died two weeks before, and he could not understand why he was not over it yet. He had no experience or information about the grieving process; no one had told him that it would take many more than two weeks to mourn his beloved grandmother.

Sometimes even healthy grief is mistaken for a kind of illness or a sign of depression that must be immediately remedied. But grief is not something to fix. It is a response to love and loss. When someone you love deeply dies, over the coming years you learn that grief does not go away, it becomes something you live with. But grieving, especially the early intense years, creates a social disorientation. The rest of the world is busily moving on about their business as if nothing has happened. But, for me, the earth had shifted on its axis, and everything had happened, shifted, changed. Many people, especially those unfamiliar with grief, wish that you would just get on with life.

It is at this point that attending a grief support group is incredibly helpful for many people, including me. It is an unusual experience of heading down to a church basement or into a conference room at a hospice or a hospital meeting room. You meet weekly with complete strangers with whom you may have absolutely nothing in common except for the huge grief that you carry with you, which is everything at that moment.

Hospice and other grief programs in the United States have been largely supportive of including LGBT grievers, in my personal and professional experience. However, they do not necessarily address the differences that LGBT grievers undergo. Moreover, several other LGBT people who had experienced a significant loss have told me that they never considered attending a general grief support group. They were concerned that they would be refused service by the provider because of their sexual orientation or gender identity or that they would encounter prejudice (anti-LGBT or racism) within the group. These perceived barriers, based on their own previous experiences of anti-LGBT and racist attitudes by both society and health care providers, were too much to overcome in the midst of grieving.

Same-gender couples, polyamorous relationships, and partnerships that include a transgender person are still not generally accorded the same respect as heterosexual, non-transgender couples in the United States.[1] In 1989, Kenneth Doka first wrote about the concept of disenfranchised grief, in which some grievers are not given a right to grieve by society because of the type of relationship between the deceased and the griever, among other factors. He later expounds on this, noting that: "Although an individual may have an intense and multi-faceted reaction to loss, that loss and the ensuing responses may be unacknowledged by surrounding others or by society at large. Although the individual grieves, others do not acknowledge that the individual has the right to grieve. The person is not offered the 'rights' or the 'grieving role' that would lay claim to social sympathy and support or given such compensations as time off from work or diminishment of social responsibilities."[2]

Thus, a griever whose relationship is not respected will not be accorded the same respect for their grief process because of who the person is grieving or whether the relationship was considered valid. This greatly increases the sense of alienation and disorientation experienced by the griever. When the life of the deceased is devalued by society—as is experienced by people of color, those with disabilities, transgender people, people with HIV/AIDS, and more—then those who grieve them may also be devalued and disregarded. These attitudes compound the tragedy of loss and the sense of alienation.

Those who are closeted may face even deeper levels of disenfranchised grief, as those around the bereaved may not even be aware that they are grieving and are unable to correctly interpret the griever's emotional state. In one blog post about an LGBT grief support group, the author notes, "One man said that by attending our group he was 'coming out' in public for the first time. He never even took the bereavement days from his work because he was afraid to say why he needed them."[3] Imagine losing a partner or other loved one and going to work the next day pretending nothing at all had happened. In addition, being closeted or simply living in a society that does not accept us requires us to shut off aspects of ourselves; this, some experts say, must also be grieved.[4]

Even those who are out may not be acknowledged by the deceased person's family of origin. The funeral itself can be traumatic, rather than comforting. In an article on gay and lesbian grief, Dudley Cave writes, "A funeral should be a springboard for good grief, but can be a disaster for the survivor of a same-sex couple who, if not excluded by the blood relatives, can be at the back shrouded in personal grief, while all the sympathy is being directed to the family at the front. . . . Even when the relationship is fairly open and the parents appear to regard the partner as another son or daughter, they may want the relationship concealed at the funeral and even ask the partner not to attend or to act as an acquaintance only—because 'the neighbors would not understand.'"[5]

When a transgender or gender nonconforming person dies, they may be misgendered by their family of origin and funeral services conducted using the name the deceased was given at birth, rather than the name that their loved ones know and use.[6] This act of disrespect is deeply painful to friends and chosen family members. Thus, in these ways, LGBT people often begin the grieving process at a disadvantage—without social recognition of the nature or extent of the loss, without respect for the identity of the deceased, and without the same support as that received by heterosexual, gender-normative people.

Yet for many LGBT people, our relationships are a vital source of meaning and satisfaction in life. In an article based on extensive interviews with gay men, Peter Robertson notes, "The principle reason a relationship is meaningful to the men in this sample of interviewees is because it is both the central focus of their life and a project they jointly develop with their partner."[7] Vicky Whipple comments in her book on lesbian widows about the intensity of lesbian relationships, noting, "There is a sense of intimacy within lesbian relationships that is emotionally gratifying to both partners. One nationwide study indicated that 95 percent of lesbians who participated in that particular research project expressed the hope that they would grow old together with their current partner."[8] Thus, while society at large may diminish the importance of same-sex or queer intimate relationships, many within the community place tremendous value in these relationships. When one partner dies, this leads to a profound sense of loss, yet families of origin, coworkers, and others surrounding the bereaved may consciously or unconsciously minimize this loss.

This situation may be compounded for those who have experienced multiple losses as a result of the HIV/AIDS epidemic. Some grievers have previously lost a partner or partners and multiple close friends; a more recent loss reawakens grief and adds to it. Those who lived through the deadliest years of the epidemic may never have had time to adequately grieve some of their losses, since some people experienced almost continual loss. Dagmawi Woubshet powerfully argues that AIDS grief is similar to mourning experienced by the Black community: "in the insistence that death is ever present, that death is somehow always impending, and that survivors can confront all this death in the face of shame and stigma in eloquent ways that also often imply a fierce political sensibility and a longing for justice."[9] An article on multiple AIDS-related losses points out that people may need to "grieve the fact that there is so much to grieve."[10] The authors go on to note the particular importance of social support in these instances: "Those who tend to isolate themselves from others will have a much more difficult time adjusting to the loss. Thus, individuals who are grieving multiple losses should be encouraged to seek support."[11] The HIV/AIDS epidemic created particular patterns of grief within our communities that still need to be addressed.

Yet despite all these specific challenges faced by LGBT grievers and the need for connection with others in similar circumstances, it can be challenging to find a support group that addresses these needs. Very few community centers or LGBT organizations offer such groups. Writing about lesbian widows, Whipple recounts the story of "Janet," who relates, "I checked the hospitals for bereavement groups, but did not qualify as I was not a relation of Chris, just a 'friend.' I checked the

Lambda Center and nothing was offered. I checked with cancer groups and was not refused but was not really welcome to join because her death was different (a police officer shot in the line of duty). I checked with the widows' service through the Highway Patrol and got very little acknowledgement as it was not a 'real' marriage. My heartache was no different from that of a man-woman relationship, but no one wanted to recognize it as such."[12]

Similar stories are repeated in multiple books, articles, and blogs about LGBT grievers. Support groups are difficult to find but cherished when found.

I was able to access two grief support experiences at LGBT community centers. The first was a one-time offering in late November focused on getting through the upcoming holidays. The other was a two-session group with a more general theme. As brief as these experiences were, they were critical to my grieving process. In these spaces, there was so much less to explain about my loved one or about myself. I could relax and tell my unedited story without feeling a need to translate aspects of it or worry that it might make other group members uncomfortable. I did not have to pretend to be like anyone else there. But, of course, I did end up feeling a tremendous sense of commonality with the others who came. In addition, the LGBT-focused groups were well-balanced in terms of gender, which was very different than the general support groups I attended, which were almost exclusively accessed by women and had a wider age range of participants.[13]

Based on these experiences, I firmly believe that I would have benefited from participating in a longer support group that was comprised primarily or exclusively of LGBT grievers. In fact, experts assert that disenfranchised groups particularly benefit from a group experience. Eileen McKeon Pesek writes, "Disenfranchised grievers, even more than traditional grievers, need this kind of supportive atmosphere because of the isolation, loneliness, shame, and guilt they may experience. The group setting allows them to hear and identify with others' stories. Their losses, deemed less significant or appropriate in general society, can be appreciated in the group."[14] Our communities could be greatly strengthened by offering this type of support.

In particular, I would encourage LGBT community centers and other supportive organizations to explore the possibility of adding a grief support group to their lineup of programs. This might be an ongoing group or one that meets periodically. One of the challenges that providers cite in offering LGBT-specific grief programs is that there may not be enough of a need at any given moment to fill a group. I would suggest including people at different points of the grieving process to expand the number of available people. Often support groups are geared to those within a window of three to nine months following a loss, but there can be benefits to talking with those at different stages of bereavement. Periodic workshops, such as the ones I attended, are also quite valuable.

It is important to remember that communities and cultures grieve in different ways. People of color in the United States are less likely, in general, to seek bereavement support from organizations. This is, in part, because of strong community and religious ties that meet many of the needs of grievers and partly because of racism too often encountered in institutional settings.[15] Prejudice against same-gender loving people and those of different gender presentations can disrupt these conventional community and family supports, leaving the bereaved without these traditional sources of comfort. Community groups and families of choice can help close this gap, but only if they are intentional and able to provide a truly inclusive space. I would strongly urge that community organizations seek out facilitators with experience with diverse groups and skills in addressing racism within the support group setting. It is also imperative to create outreach materials that make it clear that all are truly welcome, including people of color, transgender people, bisexuals (including those with same or different gender partners), and other groups who are marginalized within many LGBT communities.

Another helpful step would be to work with community hospice and other grief programs to encourage explicit outreach to LGBT people. Offering groups that are specifically labelled as welcoming to people of all sexual orientations and gender identities would, I firmly believe, increase the number of LGBT people and allies accessing such groups. Grief counselors and programs could work to steer LGBT people toward the same groups so at least they were not the only ones in a support group. A community center, LGBT affirming community of faith, or other groups could offer to host a hospice-based program, communicating to LGBT people that the group meets in an affirming space.

It is important to remember that it may take a bereaved person some time to decide to attend a support group. It requires courage to face grief and loss; it makes us vulnerable and can be very painful, even while it is healing. This means that offering a program once is not enough; people may need to see the program listed for many months before they decide to attend. Perseverance matters.

The death of someone we love is heartbreaking, and grief lasts months and years. LGBT people may face loss without the same levels of compassion, sympathy, and support as our heterosexual, non-transgender peers, and yet we share the same human needs for comfort and healing. Evidence shows that support groups can make a significant difference for disenfranchised grievers, affirming the depths of their love and their grief. LGBT community groups can play a valuable role in increasing opportunities for LGBT grievers to meet with others who have experienced loss and are seeking healing together.

Rev. Dr. Justin Sabia-Tanis earned his PhD from the Graduate Theological Union and holds a master's degree from Harvard Divinity School and a doctorate from San Francisco Theological Seminary. His career includes pastoral ministry and nonprofit work. He is the author of *Transgender: Ministry, Theology, and Communities of Faith* and also contributed chapters to the *Queer Bible Commentary* and *Take Back the Word: A Queer Reading of the Bible*. He currently works for the Center for LGBTQ and Gender Studies in Religion and teaches at the college and seminary levels.

Notes

1 For example, while heterosexual people may agree with according legal marriage rights to same-sex couples, they remain uncomfortable with seeing evidence of affection between these couples; see Long Doan, Annalise Loehr, and Lisa R. Miller, "Formal Rights and Informal Privileges for Same-Sex Couples: Evidence from a National Survey Experiment," *American Sociological Review* 79, no. 6 (November 2014), accessed June 6, 2019, https://journals.sagepub.com/doi/10.1177/0003122414555886.

2 Kenneth J. Doka, ed., *Disenfranchised Grief: New Directions, Challenges, and Strategies for Practice* (Champaign, IL: Research Press, 2002), 6.

3 "LGBT Grief & the Importance of Finding Support," Grief in Common, September 2017, accessed June 6, 2019, http://www.griefincommon.com/blog/lgbt-grief-importance-finding-support/.

4 John E. Hart, "Gay Men: Grieving the Effects of Homophobia," in *Men Coping with Grief* (Death, Value, and Meaning Series), ed. Dale A. Lund (Amityville, NY: Baywood Publishing Company, 2000), 65. Hart goes on to describe the value of support groups in grieving and healing from internalized homophobia and

shame. This would be useful reading for those considering conducting bereavement groups for LGBTQ people.

5 Dudley Cave, "Gay and Lesbian Bereavement," in *Death, Dying and Bereavement*, 2nd edition, ed. Donna L. Dickenson (Thousand Oaks, CA: SAGE Publications, 2000), 364.

6 Kristen E. Porter, Mark Brennan-Ing, Sand C. Chang, lore m. dickey, Anneliese A. Sing, Kyle L. Bower, and Taryn M. Witten, "Providing Competent and Affirming Services for Transgender and Gender Nonconforming Older Adults," *Clinical Gerontologist* 39, no. 5 (July 2016): 377.

7 Peter Robinson, *The Changing World of Gay Men* (London: Palgrave Macmillan, 2008), 116.

8 Vicky Whipple, *Lesbian Widows: Invisible Grief* (New York: Harrington Park Press, 2006), 5–6.

9 Dagmawi Woubshet, *The Calendar of Loss: Race, Sexuality, and Mourning in the Early Era of AIDS* (Baltimore, MD: Johns Hopkins University Press, 2015), 5.

10 Carrie A. Springer and Suzanne H. Lease, "The Impact of Multiple AIDS-Related Bereavement in the Gay Male Population," *Journal of Counseling & Development* 78, no. 3 (July 2000): 301.

11 Ibid.

12 Whipple, *Lesbian Widows*, 135.

13 In the United States, women attend grief support groups in much higher numbers than men; see, e.g., Perry Garfinkel, "Men Seek Gender-Specific Bereavement Groups," *New York Times*, July 25, 2011, accessed June 6, 2019, https://www.nytimes.com/2011/07/26/health/26grief.html?mtrref=www.google.com&gwh=32D95A5C470BD98B2753F83BB6BEE3F5&gwt=pay.

14 Eileen McKeon Pesek, "The Role of Support Groups in Disenfranchised Grief," in *Disenfranchised Grief*, 133.

15 Anna Laurie and Robert A. Neimeyer, "African Americans in Bereavement: Grief as a Function of Ethnicity," *Omega* 57, no. 2 (October 2008): 175, accessed June 6, 2019, https://pdfs.semanticscholar.org/e91f/c2b03f8c113394127ea1424da9c3d7d46581.pdf?_ga=2.114528527.947130781.1559856824-1721515678.1559514554.

Conclusion

Adrian Shanker

These essays and the unheard stories of other LGBT people make it clear: LGBT people experience health challenges pervasively, throughout our bodies and throughout our lives. The question is: *What are we going to do about it?*

Will health care professionals take this information to heart, train themselves on LGBT-specific issues within their specialties and scopes of practice and make an effort to provide high-quality, culturally appropriate care for LGBT patients?

Will curricula in medical, nursing, social work, counseling, and public health programs evolve to include specific training on LGBT health?

Will policy makers prioritize historically marginalized populations, including the LGBT community, and work to enact health policy changes responsive to our community's proven needs?

Will activists organize and mobilize for queer health?

Will researchers include LGBT demographic data questions within their research projects?

If the answer to these questions is *yes*, then we can predict improvements in behavioral, clinical, and policy outcomes for LGBT consumers of health care. There is nothing biological about LGBT people to prevent health equity. Our health challenges are grounded in a history of bias, discrimination, stigma, and structural barriers to care. These are fixable problems, if we work for it.

Afterword

Kate Kendell

Throughout my career, I've been involved with some of the LGBT movement's greatest fights: marriage equality, nondiscrimination in the workplace, parenting rights, inclusion in sports, ending conversion therapy, protecting youth, elders, and LGBT families. The common thread that links all these issues is health and well-being. It is not possible to be a healthy, vital person if you are under assault for who you are. Precisely because so many LGBT individuals struggle with stigma, safety, acceptance, and belonging, many in our community still struggle with high rates of mental and physical health challenges.

Despite the odds, our movement for LGBT liberation has come far. In my twenty-two years leading the National Center for Lesbian Rights (NCLR), I had a front-row seat to our national progress. Out of nothing and in the face of hostility from our own government we built the HIV/AIDS infrastructure in the 1980s to fight back and save our men and everyone impacted by the pandemic. When I started at the NCLR in the 1990s, LGBT parents routinely lost custody of their children as they came out of heterosexual marriages. Now, sexual orientation is not a basis for losing custody. In the early 2000s, many openly wondered if we should fight for the freedom to marry or if such a fight would be successful in their lifetimes. In 2015, we won marriage nationwide at the U.S. Supreme Court.

We've come a long way from the time when LGBT people were dying left and right from a treatable virus to witnessing some of those early AIDS activists marrying longtime partners. But the LGBT community still experiences open hostility and disregard from health care professionals, some LGBT health needs are still not covered equitably by health insurers, and policy makers still sometimes lack the political will to advocate for equitable policies for our community.

From obstetricians refusing to treat lesbians, to gay men being ridiculed for wanting a prescription for pre-exposure prophylaxis (PrEP). Health care professionals can do better. Policy makers can do better. All of us can do better.

Our movement for equality, for liberation, has been breathtaking in its gains. But we still fight for our humanity, our health, and our happiness. The priority for a new generation must be the health of every one of us and the promise of a long, healthy, fully embraced life.

Kate Kendell led the National Center for Lesbian Rights, a national legal organization advancing the civil and human rights of LGBT people and their families, for twenty-two years. Kate grew up Mormon in Utah and received her JD degree from the University of Utah College of Law in 1988. After a few years as a corporate attorney she was named the first staff attorney for the American Civil Liberties Union of Utah. In 1994, she accepted the position as legal director with the National Center for Lesbian Rights and made the move to San Francisco. In 1996, Kate was named the NCLR's executive director. Under Kate's leadership the NCLR won custody and family law cases, achieved victories on behalf of LGBT athletes, won protections for LGBT students and elders, and secured asylum for over three hundred clients. The NCLR was lead on the California marriage equality case in 2008 and was later part of the team of attorneys to secure national marriage equality in the 2015 U.S. Supreme Court case Obergefell v. Hodges.

About the Editor

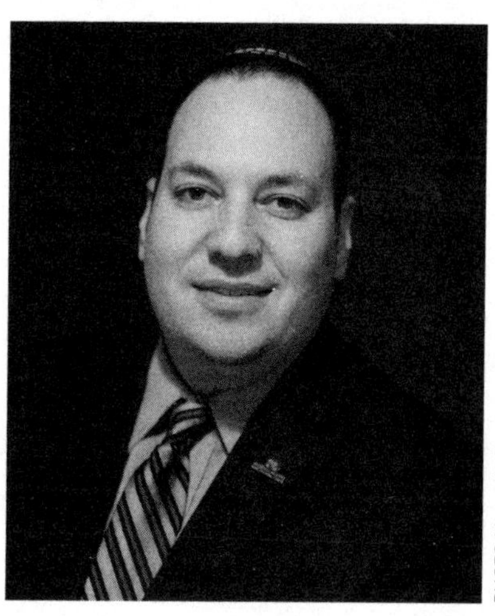
PHOTO Megan Keller

Adrian Shanker (he/him/his) is an award-winning activist and organizer whose career has centered on advancing progress for the LGBT community. He has worked as an arts fundraiser, a labor organizer, and a marketing manager, and he served as president of Equality Pennsylvania for three years before founding Bradbury-Sullivan LGBT Community Center in Allentown, Pennsylvania, where he serves as executive director.

An accomplished organizer, Adrian has led numerous successful campaigns to advance LGBT progress through municipal nondiscrimination and relationship recognition laws and laws to protect LGBT youth from conversion therapy. A specialist in LGBT health policy, he has developed leading-edge health promotion campaigns to advance health equity through behavioral, clinical, and policy changes.

Adrian administered data collection for the 2015 and 2018 Pennsylvania LGBT Health Needs Assessments. He coauthored "Queer and Quitting: Addressing Tobacco Use as an LGBTQ Issue", a chapter in *The Routledge Handbook for LGBTQIA Administration and Policy*. At the appointment of Governor Tom Wolf, he serves as a commissioner on both the Pennsylvania Commission on LGBTQ Affairs and the

Pennsylvania Human Relations Commission. Previously, he served on the Office of Health Equity Advisory Board at Pennsylvania Department of Health.

Adrian earned a Graduate Certificate in LGBT Health Policy & Practice from George Washington University and a BA *cum laude* in Political Science and Religion Studies from Muhlenberg College. Named a Healthcare Hero by *Lehigh Valley Business* and twice named Person of the Year by *Philadelphia Gay News*, Adrian has received numerous awards for his leadership, including the Bar Association of Lehigh County's Liberty Bell Award, the City of Allentown's Human Relations Award, Anne Frank Center USA's Spirit of Anne Frank Award, and GLSEN Hudson Valley's Leadership Award. He is a member of the Society for the Scientific Study of Sexuality and the Society for Public Health Educators.

About the Illustrator

Jacinta Bunnell is the author of four coloring books: *The Big Gay Alphabet Coloring Book*, *Sometimes the Spoon Runs Away with Another Spoon*, *Girls Will Be Boys Will Be Girls Will Be...* and *Girls Are Not Chicks.*

The Training Institute at Bradbury-Sullivan LGBT Community Center provides leading-edge, fully customized trainings on LGBT issues for all types of nonprofit organizations, government agencies, school districts, and businesses, with special expertise in health care, education, social and human services organizations, and law enforcement. The Training Institute also provides individualized policy development assistance for organizations seeking support with crafting LGBT-inclusive policies.

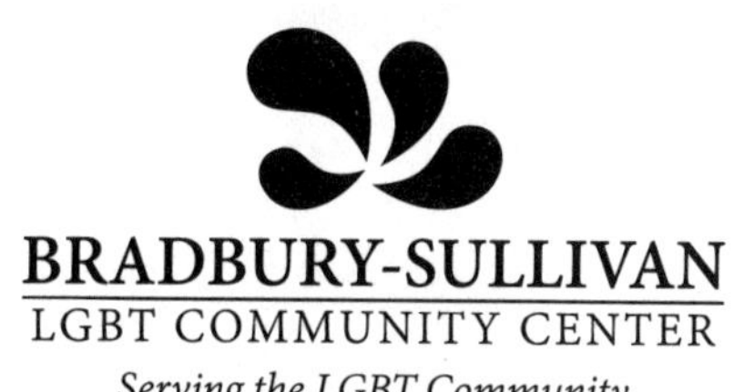

Bradbury-Sullivan LGBT Community Center produces arts, health, youth, and pride programs in Pennsylvania's Lehigh Valley region.

Headquartered in the heart of the City of Allentown, Pennsylvania, Bradbury-Sullivan LGBT Community Center provides services for urban, suburban, and rural communities. Through innovative approaches to disparity measurement, risk reduction, health promotion, and training for health professionals, Bradbury-Sullivan LGBT Community Center works on the leading edge of LGBT health and has been recognized for its model health campaigns.

Bradbury-Sullivan LGBT Community Center measures LGBT health disparities through the biannual Pennsylvania LGBT Health Needs Assessment, and then utilizes the data to develop health promotion campaigns to eliminate LGBT disparities, with a focus on tobacco, cancer, HIV, and diabetes.

Health programs at Bradbury-Sullivan LGBT Community Center have included practice-based research partnerships as part of the national discourse on LGBT health equity. In 2017, the organization was recognized with the Rural Health Program of the Year Award from the Pennsylvania Office of Rural Health.

Learn more at www.bradburysullivancenter.org

ABOUT PM PRESS

PM Press was founded at the end of 2007 by a small collection of folks with decades of publishing, media, and organizing experience. PM Press co-conspirators have published and distributed hundreds of books, pamphlets, CDs, and DVDs. Members of PM have founded enduring book fairs, spearheaded victorious tenant organizing campaigns, and worked closely with bookstores, academic conferences, and even rock bands to deliver political and challenging ideas to all walks of life. We're old enough to know what we're doing and young enough to know what's at stake.

We seek to create radical and stimulating fiction and nonfiction books, pamphlets, T-shirts, visual and audio materials to entertain, educate, and inspire you. We aim to distribute these through every available channel with every available technology—whether that means you are seeing anarchist classics at our bookfair stalls, reading our latest vegan cookbook at the café, downloading geeky fiction e-books, or digging new music and timely videos from our website.

PM Press is always on the lookout for talented and skilled volunteers, artists, activists, and writers to work with. If you have a great idea for a project or can contribute in some way, please get in touch.

PM Press
PO Box 23912
Oakland, CA 94623
www.pmpress.org

PM Press in Europe
europe@pmpress.org
www.pmpress.org.uk

FRIENDS OF PM PRESS

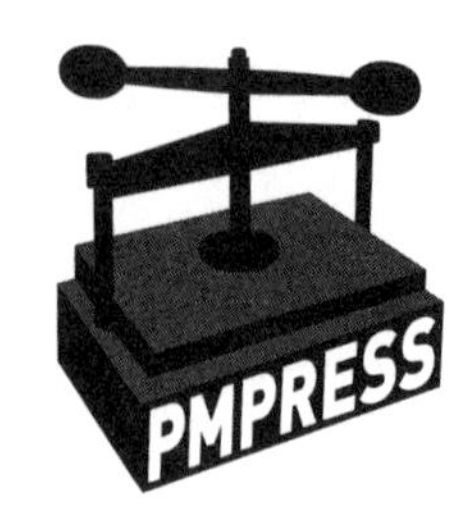

These are indisputably momentous times—the financial system is melting down globally and the Empire is stumbling. Now more than ever there is a vital need for radical ideas.

In the years since its founding—and on a mere shoestring—PM Press has risen to the formidable challenge of publishing and distributing knowledge and entertainment for the struggles ahead. With over 300 releases to date, we have published an impressive and stimulating array of literature, art, music, politics, and culture. Using every available medium, we've succeeded in connecting those hungry for ideas and information to those putting them into practice.

Friends of PM allows you to directly help impact, amplify, and revitalize the discourse and actions of radical writers, filmmakers, and artists. It provides us with a stable foundation from which we can build upon our early successes and provides a much-needed subsidy for the materials that can't necessarily pay their own way. You can help make that happen—and receive every new title automatically delivered to your door once a month—by joining as a Friend of PM Press. And, we'll throw in a free T-shirt when you sign up.

Here are your options:

- **$30 a month** Get all books and pamphlets plus 50% discount on all webstore purchases
- **$40 a month** Get all PM Press releases (including CDs and DVDs) plus 50% discount on all webstore purchases
- **$100 a month** Superstar—Everything plus PM merchandise, free downloads, and 50% discount on all webstore purchases

For those who can't afford $30 or more a month, we have **Sustainer Rates** at $15, $10 and $5. Sustainers get a free PM Press T-shirt and a 50% discount on all purchases from our website.

Your Visa or Mastercard will be billed once a month, until you tell us to stop. Or until our efforts succeed in bringing the revolution around. Or the financial meltdown of Capital makes plastic redundant. Whichever comes first.

Girls Are Not Chicks Coloring Book

Jacinta Bunnell and Julie Novak

ISBN: 978-1-60486-076-4
$10.00 36 pages

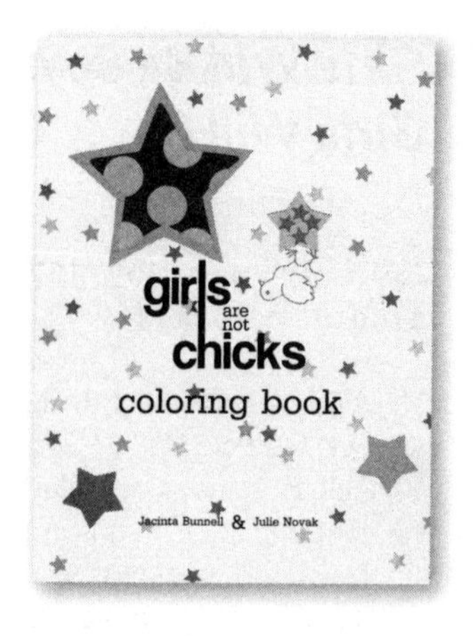

Twenty-seven pages of feminist fun! This is a coloring book you will never outgrow. *Girls Are Not Chicks* is a subversive and playful way to examine how pervasive gender stereotypes are in every aspect of our lives. This book helps to deconstruct the homogeneity of gender expression in children's media by showing diverse pictures that reinforce positive gender roles for girls.

Color the Rapunzel for a new society. She now has power tools, a roll of duct tape, a Tina Turner album, and a bus pass!

Paint outside the lines with Miss Muffet as she tells that spider off and considers a career as an arachnologist!

Girls are not chicks. Girls are thinkers, creators, fighters, healers, and superheroes.

"An ingeniously subversive coloring book."
—Heather Findlay, editor in chief, *Girlfriends* magazine

"Get this cool feminist coloring book even if you don't have a kid"
—Jane Pratt, *Jane* magazine

Girls Will Be Boys Will Be Girls Will Be . . . Coloring Book

Jacinta Bunnell

ISBN: 978-1-62963-507-1
$11.00 40 pages

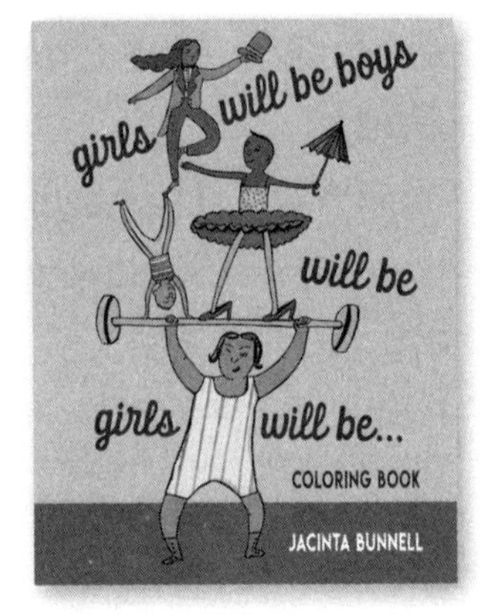

This updated edition of the iconic coloring book *Girls Will Be Boys Will Be Girls Will Be . . .* by Jacinta Bunnell contains all new illustrations and questions for contemplation. In this groundbreaking coloring book, you will meet girls who build drum sets and fix bikes, boys who bake and knit, and all manner of children along the gender spectrum. Children are tender, vulnerable, tough, zany, courageous, and gentle, no matter what their gender. This coloring book is for all the heroic handsome beauties of the world and for everyone who has ever colored outside the lines—a reminder that we never need to compromise ourselves to fit someone else's idea of who we ought to be.

Featuring illustrations by Giselle Potter, Nicole Georges, Kristine Virsis, Simi Stone, Jacinta Bunnell, Nicole Rodrigues, Richard Wentworth, and many more, this is the perfect book for the gender creative person in your life. The future is gender fabulous.

"A perfect alternative to gender-saturated Disney fare."
—*Bitch* magazine

"A great inexpensive gift for kids age 5 to 95."
—*Curve* magazine

"If I had had this coloring book when I was little, I think things would have been a little easier for me, and when you're little a little easier is a lot."
—Lynda Barry, cartoonist

Sometimes the Spoon Runs Away with Another Spoon Coloring Book

Jacinta Bunnell and Nathaniel Kusinitz

ISBN: 978-1-60486-329-1
$10.00 36 pages

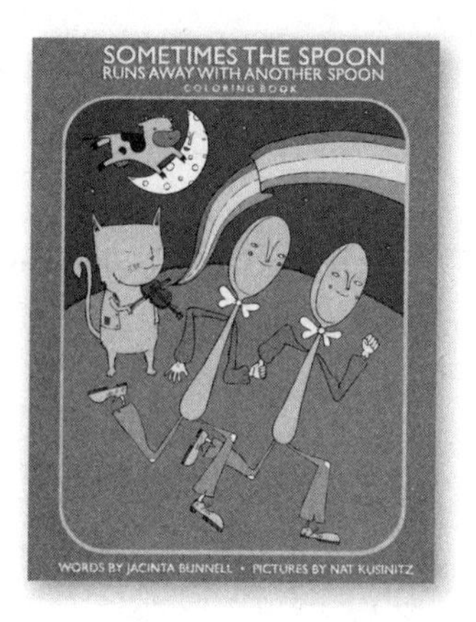

We have the power to change fairy tales and nursery rhymes so that these stories are more realistic. In *Sometimes the Spoon Runs Away With Another Spoon* you will find anecdotes of real kids' lives and true-to-life fairy tale characters. This book pushes us beyond rigid gender expectations while we color fantastic beasts who like pretty jewelry and princesses who build rocket ships.

Celebrate sensitive boys, tough girls, and others who do not fit into a disempowering gender categorization.

Sometimes the Spoon . . . aids the work of dismantling the Princess Industrial Complex by moving us forward with more honest representations of our children and ourselves. Color to your heart's content. Laugh along with the characters. Write your own fairy tales. Share your own truths.

"As moving and funny as Walter the Farting Dog, *with pictures you can color however your heart desires,* Sometimes the Spoon . . . *is appropriate for children of all ages, especially those who grew up without it."*
—Ayun Halliday, Chief Primatologist of *The East Village Inky*

"For some people the sky's the limit. For Jacinta Bunnell it's a place to put a rainbow. There are no limits in Sometimes the Spoon Runs Away With Another Spoon*—just fun and love. Jacinta Bunnell invites you to 'Step right up!' to the wonderful world of you!"*
—World Famous *BOB*, *Ultimate Self Confidence! Coach*

The Big Gay Alphabet Coloring Book

Jacinta Bunnell
Illustrated by Leela Corman

ISBN: 978-1-62963-092-2
$12.95 64 pages

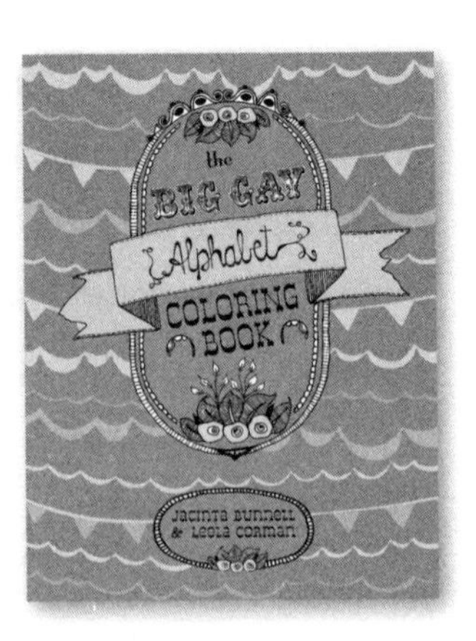

Grab your crayons and your backpack for a fantastical journey through *The Big Gay Alphabet Coloring Book*, sixty-four pages illustrating twenty-six words that highlight memorable victories and collective moments in LGBTQP (Lesbian, Gay, Bisexual, Transgender, Queer, Questioning, and Pansexual) culture.

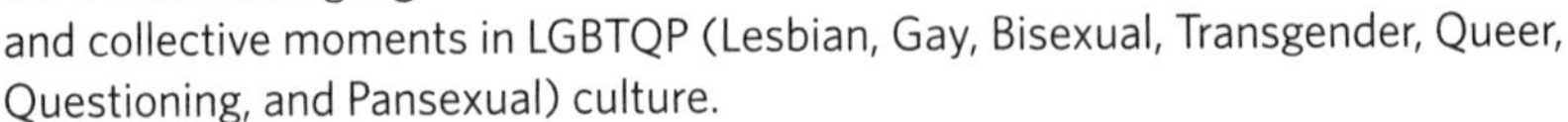

The Big Gay Alphabet Coloring Book is Jacinta Bunnell's fourth book in the Queerbook Committee series of coloring books (including *Girls Are Not Chicks* and *Sometimes the Spoon Runs Away with Another Spoon*) and the first with acclaimed illustrator Leela Corman (*Unterzakhn*). As you add your own extraordinary colors to these pages, we hope you are left asking, "Isn't everything fabulous in this world just a little bit gay?" This notion is celebrated on every unique page, made up of inked and framed line drawings with beautiful typography, reminiscent of a handsomely designed vintage children's alphabet book.

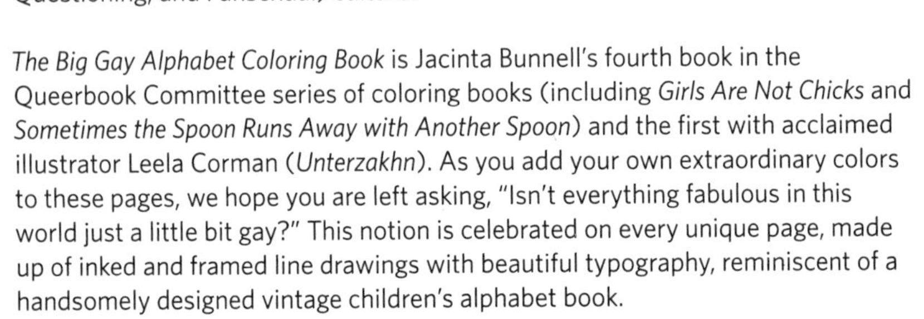

Each day, we take another step toward a greater understanding of gender fluidity, gender diversity, and sexual orientation. Change does not come easily or unfold overnight. But together we are an unflappable squad of comrades staring down oppression while stopping to make art and find joy along the way.

"With beautifully rendered moments of Queer life, The Big Gay Alphabet Coloring Book *offers over fifty pages of inked and framed line drawings and typography for folks of all ages, a tool for education and inspiration."*
—Cristy C. Road, author and illustrator of *Spit and Passion*

"Two of my favorite people in the world also happen to be among the most talented. I will add it to my new-parent gift pack, alongside Bunnell's other coloring book projects."
—Anne Elizabeth Moore, The Ladydrawers Comics Collective

"Jacinta and Leela have created a beautiful, fun coloring book which teaches us that everyone is deserving of respect and understanding. I'm only halfway into this thing and I've already gone through three tubes of glitter!"
—Jon Wurster, Bob Mould Band

Health Care Revolt: How to Organize, Build a Health Care System, and Resuscitate Democracy—All at the Same Time

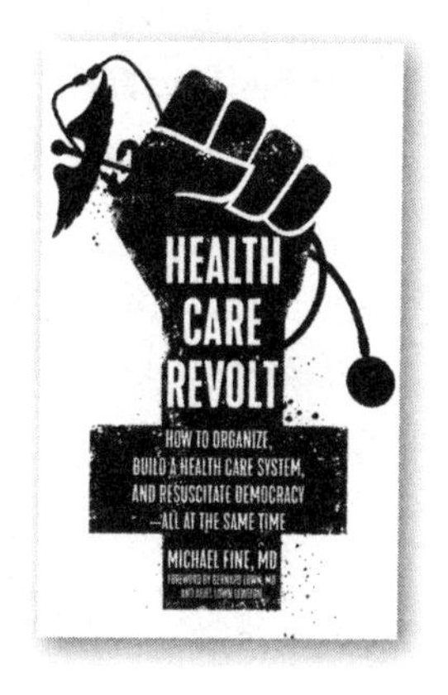

Michael Fine with a Foreword by Bernard Lown and Ariel Lown Lewiton

ISBN: 978-1-62963-581-1
$15.95 192 pages

The U.S. does not have a health system. Instead we have market for health-related goods and services, a market in which the few profit from the public's ill-health.

Health Care Revolt looks around the world for examples of health care systems that are effective and affordable, pictures such a system for the U.S., and creates a practical playbook for a political revolution in health care that will allow the nation to protect health while strengthening democracy.

Dr. Fine writes with the wisdom of a clinician, the savvy of a state public health commissioner, the precision of a scholar, and the energy and commitment of a community organizer.

"This is a revolutionary book. The author incites readers to embark on an audacious revolution to convert the American medical market into the American health care system."
—T.P. Gariepy, Stonehill College/CHOICE connect

"Michael Fine is one of the true heroes of primary care over several decades."
—Dr. Doug Henley, CEO and executive vice president of the American Academy of Family Physicians

"As Rhode Island's director of health, Dr. Fine brought a vision of a humane, local, integrated health care system that focused as much on health as on disease and treatment."
—U.S. Senator Sheldon Whitehouse

"Michael Fine has given us an extraordinary biopic on health care in America based on the authority of his forty-year career as writer, community organizer, family physician, and public health official."
—Fitzhugh Mullan, MD

Revolutionary Mothering: Love on the Front Lines

Edited by Alexis Pauline Gumbs, China Martens, and Mai'a Williams with a preface by Loretta J. Ross

ISBN: 978-1-62963-110-3
$17.95 272 pages

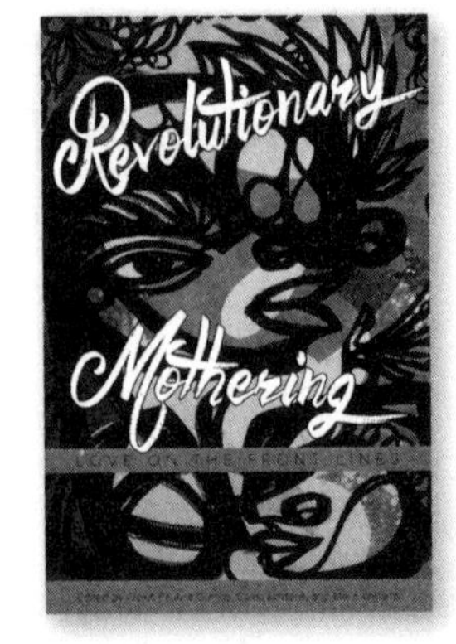

Inspired by the legacy of radical and queer black feminists of the 1970s and '80s, *Revolutionary Mothering* places marginalized mothers of color at the center of a world of necessary transformation. The challenges we face as movements working for racial, economic, reproductive, gender, and food justice, as well as anti-violence, anti-imperialist, and queer liberation are the same challenges that many mothers face every day. Oppressed mothers create a generous space for life in the face of life-threatening limits, activate a powerful vision of the future while navigating tangible concerns in the present, move beyond individual narratives of choice toward collective solutions, live for more than ourselves, and remain accountable to a future that we cannot always see. *Revolutionary Mothering* is a movement-shifting anthology committed to birthing new worlds, full of faith and hope for what we can raise up together.

Contributors include June Jordan, Malkia A. Cyril, Esteli Juarez, Cynthia Dewi Oka, Fabiola Sandoval, Sumayyah Talibah, Victoria Law, Tara Villalba, Lola Mondragón, Christy NaMee Eriksen, Norma Angelica Marrun, Vivian Chin, Rachel Broadwater, Autumn Brown, Layne Russell, Noemi Martinez, Katie Kaput, alba onofrio, Gabriela Sandoval, Cheryl Boyce Taylor, Ariel Gore, Claire Barrera, Lisa Factora-Borchers, Fabielle Georges, H. Bindy K. Kang, Terri Nilliasca, Irene Lara, Panquetzani, Mamas of Color Rising, tk karakashian tunchez, Arielle Julia Brown, Lindsey Campbell, Micaela Cadena, and Karen Su.

"This collection is a treat for anyone that sees class and that needs to learn more about the experiences of women of color (and who doesn't?!). There is no dogma here, just fresh ideas and women of color taking on capitalism, anti-racist, anti-sexist theory-building that is rooted in the most primal of human connections, the making of two people from the body of one: mothering."
—Barbara Jensen, author of *Reading Classes: On Culture and Classism in America*

"For women of color, mothering—the art of mothering—has been framed by the most virulent systems, historically: enslavement, colonialism, capitalism, imperialism. We have had few opportunities to define mothering not only as an aspect of individual lives and choices, but as the processes of love and as a way of structuring community. Revolutionary Mothering *arrives as a needed balm."*
—Alexis De Veaux, author of *Warrior Poet: A Biography of Audre Lorde*

Speaking OUT: Queer Youth in Focus

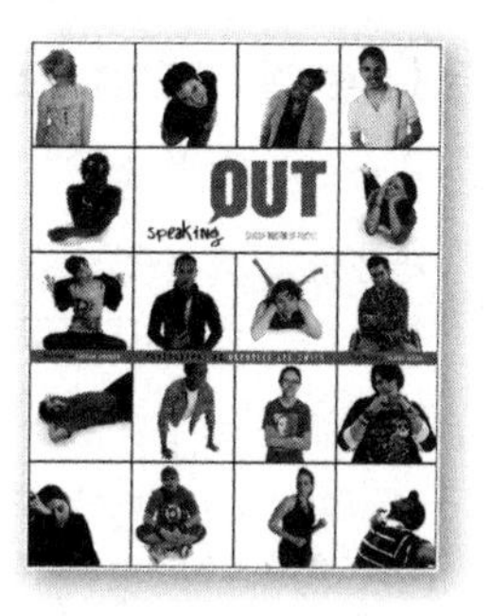

Rachelle Lee Smith, with a foreword by Candace Gingrich and an afterword by Graeme Taylor

ISBN: 978-1-62963-041-0
$14.95 128 pages

Speaking OUT: Queer Youth in Focus is a photographic essay that explores a wide spectrum of experiences told from the perspective of a diverse group of young people, ages fourteen to twenty-four, identifying as queer (i.e., lesbian, gay, bisexual, transgender, or questioning). Portraits are presented without judgment or stereotype by eliminating environmental influence with a stark white backdrop. This backdrop acts as a blank canvas, where each subject's personal thoughts are handwritten onto the final photographic print. With more than sixty-five portraits photographed over a period of ten years, *Speaking OUT* provides rare insight into the passions, confusions, prejudices, joys, and sorrows felt by queer youth.

Speaking OUT gives a voice to an underserved group of people that are seldom heard and often silenced. The collaboration of image and first-person narrative serves to provide an outlet, show support, create dialogue, and help those who struggle. It not only shows unity within the LGBTQ community, but also commonalities regardless of age, race, gender, and sexual orientation.

With recent media attention and the success of initiatives such as the It Gets Better Project, resources for queer youth have grown. Still, a void exists which *Speaking OUT* directly addresses: this book is for youth, by youth.

Speaking OUT is an award-winning, nationally and internationally shown and published body of work. These images have been published in magazines such as the *Advocate*, *School Library Journal*, *Curve*, *Girlfriends*, and *Out*, and showcased by the Human Rights Campaign, National Public Radio, Public Television, and the U.S. Department of Education. The work continues to show in galleries, universities, youth centers, and churches around the world.

"Rachelle Lee Smith has created a book that is not only visually stunning but also gripping with powerful words and even more inspiring young people! This is an important work of art! I highly recommend buying it and sharing it!"
—Perez Hilton, blogger and television personality

"It's often said that our youth are our future. In the LGBT community, before they become the future we must help them survive today. This book showcases the diversity of creative imagination it takes to get us to tomorrow."
—Mark Segal, award-winning LGBT journalist

The Beatrix Gates

Rachel Pollack

ISBN: 978-1-62963-578-1
$14.00 128 pages

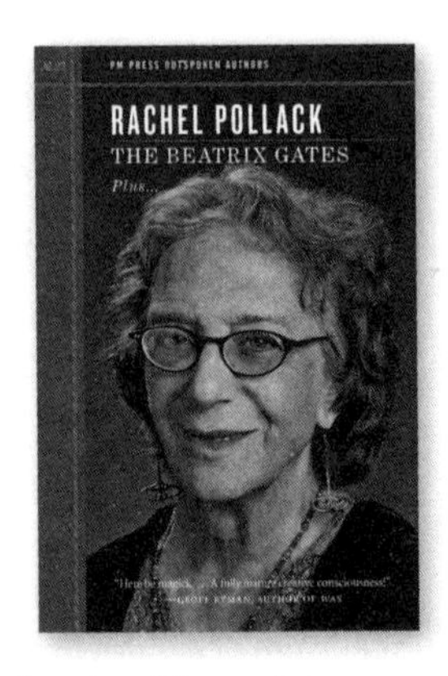

Rachel Pollack is a sorceress, a wizard with words who spins together the spiritual, the political, and the passionate in her unique, indeed inimitable, tales. An award-winning SF and Fantasy author, she is also an esteemed Tarot Grand Master with devotees and students around the world. A progressive voice in the transgender community and a trusted guide to the ancient traditions of shamanism, she writes of shimmering and dangerous worlds that have never been imagined before—much less explored. Her queer cult favorite "The Beatrix Gates" draws on magic realism, quantum science, memoir, and myth to tell the story of a girl born not in the wrong body but in the wrong universe.

Plus... "Trans Central Station," written especially for this volume, is Pollack's personal and penetrating take on the transgender experience then and now—and tomorrow? "Burning Beard" is a fiercely revisionist Old Testament tale of plague and prophecy told through a postmodern prose of, shall we say, many colors. "The Woman Who Didn't Come Back" is about just what it says it's about.

And Featuring: Our Outspoken Interview, which tells us all about comics history, the automotive origins of Tarot, the benefits of Nerd celebrity, and why the Sun exists. It will be on the test.

"Rachel Pollack's The Beatrix Gates *is a marvelous example of how sci-fi can remythologize the terms of common experience to elucidate and give new and deeper meaning."*
—Lambda Book Report

"The Beatrix Gates *is a stunning study in identity and mutability. It can be read most easily as a story about transexualism or simply a powerful examination of difference and its more positive consequences, as well as a subtle investigation of exactly what makes our identities."*
—Green Man Review

"One of the most gifted and sensitive fantasists working today."
—Publishers Weekly

"Rachel Pollack is one of the most consistently interesting and individual writers working in the fantasy and science fiction slipstream. Here be magick, real people, alternative worlds, and a fully mature creative consciousness."
—Geoff Ryman, author of *WAS*

All of Me: Stories of Love, Anger, and the Female Body

Edited by Dani Burlison

ISBN: 978-1-62963-705-1
$19.95 240 pages

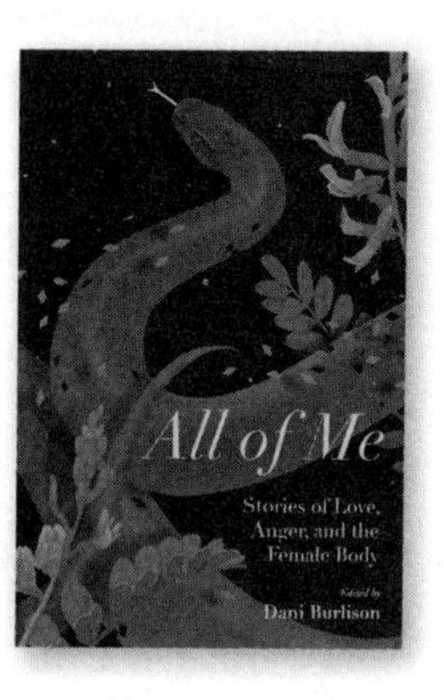

With women's anger, empowerment, and the critical importance of intersectional feminism taking center stage in much of the dialogue happening in feminist spaces right now, an anthology like this has never been more important. The voices in this collection of essays and interviews offer perspectives and experiences that help women find common ground, unity, and allyship.

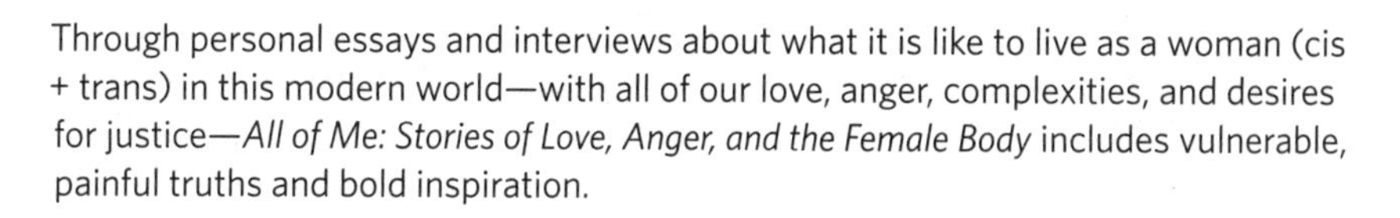
Through personal essays and interviews about what it is like to live as a woman (cis + trans) in this modern world—with all of our love, anger, complexities, and desires for justice—*All of Me: Stories of Love, Anger, and the Female Body* includes vulnerable, painful truths and bold inspiration.

This anthology is for seasoned feminists and young feminists alike—anyone looking to find inspiration in radical activism, creativity, healing, and more. This book covers topics of social and economic justice, creativity, racism, transgender perspectives, sexuality, sex work, addiction and recovery, reproductive rights, assault, relationship dynamics, families, fitting and not fitting in, radical self-care, witchcraft, and more.

If love and anger are two sides of the same coin, for women there are worlds to be explored with every flip of that coin. Readers will find a glimpse into those worlds in the pages of *All of Me*.

Contributors include Silvia Federici, Michelle Cruz Gonzales, Ariel Gore, Laurie Penny, Lidia Yuknavitch, Christine No, Kandis Williams, Vatan Doost, Deya, Phoenix LeFae, Anna Silastre, Michel Wing, Bethany Ridenour, Lorelle Saxena, Airial Clark, Patty Stonefish, Nayomi Munaweera, Melissa Madera, Margaret Elysia Garcia, Leilani Clark, Ariel Erskine, Wendy-O Matik, Kara Vernor, Starhawk, adrienne maree brown, Gerri Ravyn Stanfield, Sanam Mahloudji, Melissa Chadburn, Avery Erickson, and Milla Prince.

"Visceral, raw, and personal, All of Me *is the barbaric yawp of womanhood unrestrained. Ranging from the confessional to the call to action, this collection of deeply personal writings tears back the veil of womanhood to show the glorious and gritty guts of it all. Unfiltered, unadulterated, open; witness the wounds and the wisdom of what it means to be a woman today."*
—Lasara Firefox Allen, author of *Jailbreaking the Goddess: A Radical Revisioning of Feminist Spirituality*

Rad Families: A Celebration

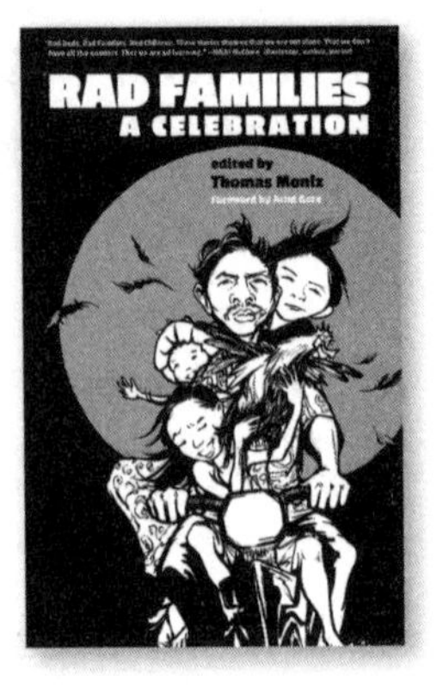

Edited by Tomas Moniz
with a Foreword by Ariel Gore

ISBN: 978-1-62963-230-8
$19.95 296 pages

Rad Families: A Celebration honors the messy, the painful, the playful, the beautiful, the myriad ways we create families. This is not an anthology of experts, or how-to articles on perfect parenting; it often doesn't even try to provide answers. Instead, the writers strive to be honest and vulnerable in sharing their stories and experiences, their failures and their regrets.

Gathering parents and writers from diverse communities, it explores the process of getting pregnant from trans birth to adoption, grapples with issues of racism and police brutality, probes raising feminists and feminist parenting. It plumbs the depths of empty nesting and letting go.

Some contributors are recognizable authors and activists but most are everyday parents working and loving and trying to build a better world one diaper change at a time. It's a book that reminds us all that we are not alone, that community can help us get through the difficulties, can, in fact, make us better people. It's a celebration, join us!

Contributors include Jonas Cannon, Ian MacKaye, Burke Stansbury, Danny Goot, Simon Knaphus, Artnoose, Welch Canavan, Daniel Muro LaMere, Jennifer Lewis, Zach Ellis, Alicia Dornadic, Jesse Palmer, Mindi J., Carla Bergman, Tasnim Nathoo, Rachel Galindo, Robert Liu-Trujillo, Dawn Caprice, Shawn Taylor, D.A. Begay, Philana Dollin, Airial Clark, Allison Wolfe, Roger Porter, cubbie rowland-storm, Annakai & Rob Geshlider, Jeremy Adam Smith, Frances Hardinge, Jonathan Shipley, Bronwyn Davies Glover, Amy Abugo Ongiri, Mike Araujo, Craig Elliott, Eleanor Wohlfeiler, Scott Hoshida, Plinio Hernandez, Madison Young, Nathan Torp, Sasha Vodnik, Jessie Susannah, Krista Lee Hanson, Carvell Wallace, Dani Burlison, Brian Whitman, scott winn, Kermit Playfoot, Chris Crass, and Zora Moniz.

"Rad dads, rad families, rad children. These stories show us that we are not alone. That we don't have all the answers. That we are all learning."
—Nikki McClure, illustrator, author, parent

"Rad Families *is the collection for all families."*
—Innosanto Nagara, author/illustrator of *A Is for Activist*

"This collection takes the anaesthetized myth of parenting and reminds us what intimacy looks like. . . . The contributors describe the contours of family in a way that resonates."
—Virgie Tovar, editor of *Hot & Heavy: Fierce Fat Girls on Life, Love & Fashion*

Resistance Behind Bars: The Struggles of Incarcerated Women

Victoria Law with an Introduction by Laura Whitehorn

ISBN: 978-1-60486-583-7
$20.00 320 pages

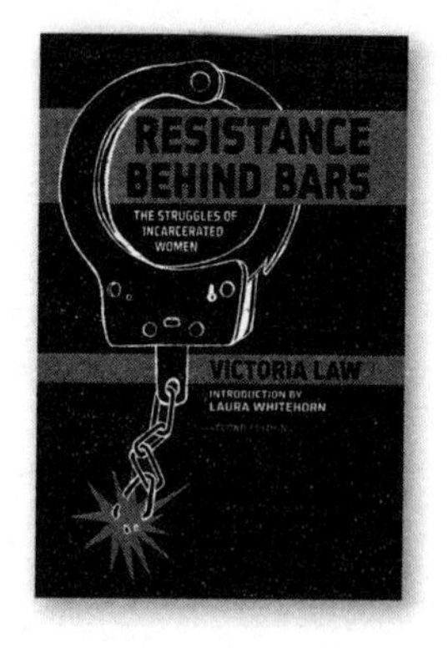

In 1974, women imprisoned at New York's maximum-security prison at Bedford Hills staged what is known as the August Rebellion. Protesting the brutal beating of a fellow prisoner, the women fought off guards, holding seven of them hostage, and took over sections of the prison.

While many have heard of the 1971 Attica prison uprising, the August Rebellion remains relatively unknown even in activist circles. *Resistance Behind Bars* is determined to challenge and change such oversights. As it examines daily struggles against appalling prison conditions and injustices, *Resistance* documents both collective organizing and individual resistance among women incarcerated in the U.S. Emphasizing women's agency in resisting the conditions of their confinement through forming peer education groups, clandestinely arranging ways for children to visit mothers in distant prisons and raising public awareness about their lives, *Resistance* seeks to spark further discussion and research into the lives of incarcerated women and galvanize much-needed outside support for their struggles.

This updated and revised edition of the 2009 PASS Award winning book includes a new chapter about transgender, transsexual, intersex, and gender-variant people in prison.

"Victoria Law's eight years of research and writing, inspired by her unflinching commitment to listen to and support women prisoners, has resulted in an illuminating effort to document the dynamic resistance of incarcerated women in the United States."
—Roxanne Dunbar-Ortiz

"Written in regular English, rather than academese, this is an impressive work of research and reportage"
—Mumia Abu-Jamal, death row political prisoner and author of *Live From Death Row*

"Finally! A passionately and extensively researched book that recognizes the myriad ways in which women resist in prison, and the many particular obstacles that, at many points, hinder them from rebelling. Even after my own years inside, I learned from this book."
—Laura Whitehorn, former political prisoner

Witches, Witch-Hunting, and Women

Silvia Federici

ISBN: 978-1-62963-568-2
$14.00 120 pages

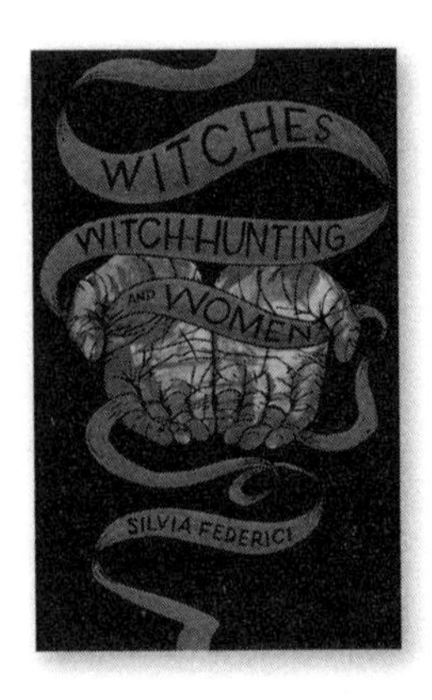

We are witnessing a new surge of interpersonal and institutional violence against women, including new witch hunts. This surge of violence has occurred alongside an expansion of capitalist social relations. In this new work that revisits some of the main themes of *Caliban and the Witch*, Silvia Federici examines the root causes of these developments and outlines the consequences for the women affected and their communities. She argues that, no less than the witch hunts in sixteenth- and seventeenth-century Europe and the "New World," this new war on women is a structural element of the new forms of capitalist accumulation. These processes are founded on the destruction of people's most basic means of reproduction. Like at the dawn of capitalism, what we discover behind today's violence against women are processes of enclosure, land dispossession, and the remolding of women's reproductive activities and subjectivity.

As well as an investigation into the causes of this new violence, the book is also a feminist call to arms. Federici's work provides new ways of understanding the methods in which women are resisting victimization and offers a powerful reminder that reconstructing the memory of the past is crucial for the struggles of the present.

"It is good to think with Silvia Federici, whose clarity of analysis and passionate vision come through in essays that chronicle enclosure and dispossession, witch-hunting and other assaults against women, in the present, no less than the past. It is even better to act armed with her insights."
—Eileen Boris, Hull Professor of Feminist Studies, University of California, Santa Barbara

"Silvia Federici's new book offers a brilliant analysis and forceful denunciation of the violence directed towards women and their communities. Her focus moves between women criminalized as witches both at the dawn of capitalism and in contemporary globalization. Federici has updated the material from her well-known book Caliban and the Witch *and brings a spotlight to the current resistance and alternatives being pursued by women and their communities through struggle."*
—Massimo De Angelis, professor of political economy, University of East London